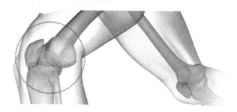

Rheumatoid
Arthritis

Other self-help guides
by How To Books

Neck and Back Pain
Dr Chris Jenner

Fibromyalgia and Myofascial Pain Syndrome
Dr Chris Jenner

Arthritis
Dr Chris Jenner

Rheumatoid Arthritis

A self-help
guide to
getting on
with your life

Jasmine Jenkins

howtobooks

An **Expert Patient** Guide

Published by How To Books Ltd,
Spring Hill House, Spring Hill Road,
Begbroke, Oxford OX5 1RX, United Kingdom.
Tel: (01865) 375794. Fax: (01865) 379162.
info@howtobooks.co.uk
www.howtobooks.co.uk

How To Books greatly reduce the carbon footprint of their books by sourcing their typesetting and printing in the UK.

First edition 2005
Second edition 2009
Third edition 2011

British Library Cataloguing in Publication Data
A catalogue record for this book is available from the British Library

ISBN 978 1 84528 463 3

Cover design by Baseline Arts Ltd, Oxford
Produced for How To Books by Deer Park Productions, Tavistock
Typeset by PDQ Typesetting Ltd, Newcastle-under-Lyme, Staffs.
Printed and bound in Great Britain by Bell & Bain Ltd, Glasgow

NOTE: The material contained in this book is set out in good faith for general guidance and no liability can be accepted for loss or expense incurred as a result of relying in particular circumstances on statements made in the book. The laws and regulations are complex and liable to change, and readers should check the current position with the relevant authorities before making personal arrangements.

Contents

Acknowledgements

I would like to thank Sue Morris for reading the text and giving me some very helpful suggestions. I would also like to thank Lynette Hartgill for doing the illustrations at such short notice. I am grateful to Dr Adam Young, my rheumatologist, for taking the time to read my book and ensuring that the medical information is accurate. He has also written a foreword for me.

A special thank you goes to Marian Ferguson for helping me to manage my rheumatoid arthritis and also for inspiring me to become an occupational therapist in the process. Finally I would like to thank Keith, my husband, as well as Carolyn, Sonia and Alison who encouraged me and supported me in writing this book as well as helping out with the editing.

Preface

This third edition is an easily readable, self-help guide for everyone with rheumatoid arthritis (RA), particularly those who are newly diagnosed. It is also useful for family carers, those working in the caring professions and health and social care students. In this new edition there are a few additions and changes as follows.

I have added in the new drugs that have become available since the last edition. There are still some new types of medication undergoing trials and it is important that people with RA contact the National Rheumatoid Arthritis Society (NRAS) by telephone or by using their website in order to keep informed.

I have also added a new chapter called Complementary Approaches in order to include some extra information on food, supplements and other complementary therapies. There is growing research in this field and I am hopeful that one day more of these therapies will be funded by the NHS. I have included the treatments that seem to be the most beneficial.

While I was thinking about what would be most useful for this new edition I came up with the idea of adding a new section of helpful suggestions and tips. I am grateful to the members of NRAS for their many suggestions and I have included these tips along with my own ideas.

Recently there has been a lot of discussion around the proposed changes to the disability employment benefits and other disability benefits like the Disability Living Allowance (DLA). I have therefore updated the disability benefits information to include some information on these latest changes.

Many of the contact details have gone out of date in the years since the last edition was published and I have therefore updated the contact details and added some new ones.

Apart from these new updates the format remains the same and I hope that it helps you to become an expert on rheumatoid arthritis.

Foreword

There have been some major changes and initiatives in the last few years in the management of rheumatoid arthritis. Some of these have been in a better understanding of the underlying mechanisms of inflammation and the development of new and effective drugs. Another very important area has been the opportunity for great patient and patient–carer involvement. Patient-led organisations have become a vital and driving force to improve the level of government funding for care of patients with rheumatoid arthritis in an ever increasing and competitive arena of health care.

Rheumatoid arthritis is a complex condition and its effects vary considerably from patient to patient. It can last for decades, and best and possible therapies are continually changing. This book covers such an important aspect of the care of rheumatoid arthritis. It reflects the need for greater input from both patients and their carers. It is unique in that a highly trained occupational therapist offers her experience both as a patient and as a therapist in what to expect and how to cope with this condition. Patients, their relatives and carers, and therapists in training, will find this account very readable. It is illuminating, sensitive and reassuring. It comes at a most opportune time.

Adam Young FRCP
Consultant Rheumatologist

Introduction

Over 30 years ago, I visited my doctor. I had severe pain in my fingers, toes and wrists. The doctor gave me anti-inflammatory drugs but he gave me no indication at all of what was wrong. These attacks occurred three more times during the next ten years; each relapse happening when each of my three daughters was three months old. I was still not aware of why all this was happening and I still received anti-inflammatory medication and no explanation.

Ten years later I visited my doctor because I couldn't understand why I had no movement in my wrist. I wanted to discover the reason for this and find out what I could do about it. I became more assertive and asked for an explanation for these attacks. Finally I was given a blood test and a referral to the consultant rheumatologist who consequently informed me that I had rheumatoid arthritis (RA). This was a devastating situation. I was 32 and I had three small children. I also had virtually no wrist movement and the joints in my fingers, toes and elbows were damaged. I was given a referral to the Occupational Therapy (OT) department. At that time I had not heard of Occupational Therapy but I decided to attend hoping that it might prove useful. I did not know then what a prominent part it would play in my life subsequently.

At the Occupational Therapy department I learnt all about my condition and how to look after my joints. I learnt exercises to improve my strength and to maintain the movements of my finger joints. I began to understand the importance of posture and how to problem solve. I was given equipment for the kitchen and I was able to discuss any problems that I had in my everyday life and find practical solutions to them. The OT department made an impression on me. I enjoyed the calmness and the time that I was given for discussion as well as the practical help that I received.

I wanted to find out more about the therapist's role in other areas of disability and I wanted to find out how to qualify. Eventually I started work as an OT assistant and later on I trained to become a fully qualified Occupational Therapist. At the time that I commenced training I was 40 and I had had rheumatoid arthritis for 18 years. It was a positive outcome from a very negative situation. I write this book from the perspective of practitioner and patient in the hope that it will enable others to gain a more positive outlook.

What is Rheumatoid Arthritis?

To know the disease is the commencement of the cure.

I am sure many readers are only too familiar with explanations about rheumatoid arthritis (RA). Nevertheless I feel that I need to explain about it to those people who are newly diagnosed or those who have not encountered the disease first hand.

Rheumatoid arthritis is a disease that occurs all over the world. The National Rheumatoid Arthritis Society[1] confirms that at present 0.8% of the adult population of the UK has rheumatoid arthritis (NRAS, 2006). This is approximately 387,000 people. The Arthritis Care booklet on rheumatoid arthritis tells us that one to three people in every hundred develop rheumatoid arthritis (Arthritis Care, 2008).[2] There are more females with the disease than males and onset is often between 30 and 55, although it can occur at any age. A study in 1999[3] stated, 'Rheumatoid arthritis is rarely seen as a serious public health issue, yet it is the single largest cause of disability in the UK.'

There is no known cause for rheumatoid arthritis and it is not directly inherited, although some predisposing factors may be. This means that it is likely that a genetic trait is then triggered by other factors like an infection, or a chemical in food, or an injury, or stress or any other as yet unknown trigger. Maybe two or three triggers are needed together, no one really knows. All that is known is that rheumatoid arthritis is an autoimmune disease. This means that the immune system is faulty and does not behave in the way that it should.

The immune system

The immune system is an intricate mechanism that enables our body to defend itself against bacteria, viruses and other organisms that want to invade it. A healthy immune system knows which particles are foreign to the body and which ones belong. In order to protect the body it will attack outsiders that do not belong. The body also protects itself when there is damage caused by an accident resulting in a burn or a broken bone. In this case inflammation occurs as a necessary part of the repair process. In rheumatoid arthritis something goes wrong and the immune system attacks its own joints.

The function of the joint

In order to understand what happens when rheumatoid arthritis attacks the joints it is first necessary to understand a little about what a joint is and what its function in the body is. I have drawn a picture of a simple joint to show what a joint looks like and what it consists of (see Figure 1). Joints can be simple, as in the elbow joint which only has movement in one direction, or complex as in the shoulder, a joint that can be moved in many ways. In any case, joints are always found at the point where different bones meet so that the bones on either side of the joint can move independently. For example, there is a joint between the upper arm bone (humerus) and the lower bones of the arm (radius/ulna bones) so that we can move the lower part of the arm independently from the upper arm. The cartilage and fluid act as a shock absorber between the bones and this helps to protect them.

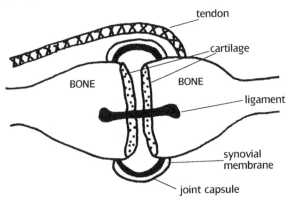

Fig. 1. Synovial joint.

How rheumatoid arthritis affects the joint

During a flare-up of rheumatoid arthritis the synovial lining of the joint becomes inflamed although it is not known what triggers the inflammation. The synovial fluid that lubricates the joint, keeping the cartilage slippery, is overproduced. The lining of the joint becomes thicker and the cartilage is destroyed. The cartilage normally acts as a shock absorber between the bones, so there will be more pain on movement when it is destroyed. Eventually if it is all destroyed the bones will fuse together, preventing the joint from working at all. Even if the bones do not fuse together the increased amount of fluid in and around the joint means that the joints become swollen and feel uncomfortable. This restricts movement at the joints even before actual damage occurs. The joint capsule and ligaments also become stretched and loose and this leads to unstable joints and deformities.

Rheumatoid arthritis and osteoarthritis: the differences

I have found that many people confuse osteoarthritis and rheumatoid arthritis. Although they both cause damage to joints the damage occurs for different reasons. Rheumatoid arthritis differs from osteoarthritis (OA) because in rheumatoid arthritis it is the faulty immune system that causes inflammation, whereas in osteoarthritis the joints become damaged through wear and tear (although inflammation may still occur). This means that osteoarthritis normally starts later in life than rheumatoid arthritis although osteoarthritis may start at 40. (People with rheumatoid arthritis may also have osteoarthritis.) In rheumatoid arthritis the joint damage is usually symmetrical but in osteoarthritis it normally is not. Another difference is that some rheumatoid arthritis sufferers may feel tired or have a feeling of being generally unwell when the inflammation occurs. In rheumatoid arthritis it is also possible to have inflammation in other organs as well as the joints, for example, the lungs and blood vessels, but usually it is the joints that are affected.

The importance of an early diagnosis

It is important to go to the doctor and obtain a diagnosis as early as possible if joint pain occurs because, as explained previously, untreated inflammation can lead to joint destruction and deformities. The early signs of rheumatoid arthritis are usually:

- pain or discomfort in the fingers or feet; and
- early morning stiffness.

The stiffness makes the limbs feel heavy and the joints feel puffy, movement becomes sluggish and it is more difficult to move the joints at all. The stiffness tends to reduce when the joints are gently moved. The disease often progresses intermittently with:

- *relapses* – when the symptoms occur;
- and *remissions* (when the symptoms stop for a period of time).

Occasionally the disease can occur rapidly with extensive pain in many joints.

The diagnosis will be done by taking a history of signs and symptoms from the client and performing a blood test, both of which are essential for the diagnosis. The development of the disease will vary from person to person. According to the Arthritis Research Campaign (ARC)[4] 20% of people with rheumatoid arthritis will have a very mild form with no damage or very minimal damage to their joints. Most people will have damage to some joints and about 5% will have a severe form of the disease with extensive joint damage and quite often some inflammation in other organs of the body too. Many people will have periods of remission when they will experience no signs of the disease. Early treatment and some adaptations to lifestyle should minimise joint damage and the effects that the disease has on everyday life.

In my own case I was not told that I had rheumatoid arthritis although I am sure the doctor would have known. Possibly he thought that it would be depressing for me to know that I had a long-term and deteriorating (chronic) condition and that I might do better without the knowledge. The problem was that I had no medication to slow the disease down and I had no therapy or guidance to tell me that I was probably making my condition worse by carrying on and ignoring it. Of course it did actually go away for four years but with rheumatoid arthritis you can never tell when it is going to return.

The unpredictability of rheumatoid arthritis

One of the main problems of the disease is its unpredictability. Even in a period of active disease it will vary from day to day and it is not often possible to know why. It could be the weather, the amount of stress on a joint, diet, an infection or any other as yet unknown factor. Research has been undertaken in order to understand the triggers of rheumatoid arthritis onset and flare-ups. However there do not appear to be any very conclusive answers.

Rheumatoid arthritis and the weather

As far as the weather goes, many people claim to feel worse in hot weather or wet weather or at the onset of a rainy period. A study by Dr Hollander in Philadelphia[5] discovered that rapid changes in barometric pressure occurring within 6–12 hours caused a greater increase in symptoms for rheumatoid arthritis patients than slower changes over 24 hours. He claims that there is no other evidence to support any other effects of the weather in exacerbating or reducing symptoms. In my own case I do not feel that the weather makes much difference, although I have sometimes noticed that one foot becomes very painful when a stormy period is building up in the atmosphere.

The significance of stress

Some research has been carried out to evaluate the role of stress in rheumatoid arthritis but again no conclusions can be drawn. One study by Marcenaro *et al*[6] in Italy in 1999 claimed that macro and micro stressful life events preceded rheumatoid arthritis onset in 86% of the cases that they studied. Macro events are very significant things like a birth, death, divorce, house move, etc. Micro events are extensive small stresses that accumulate, like difficulties with work or family. Yet a study by Haller *et al* in 1997[7] produced different results. Haller stated that 'the course of rheumatoid arthritis is influenced neither by the number of life events nor by the extent of stress caused by these events'. In my own case I am open-minded but there are some indications of stressful events playing a part, as I will explain later on.

Rheumatoid arthritis and diet

The subject of diet will be discussed later but there is some evidence for eliminating certain foods. Most of the studies that I found that evaluated diet and rheumatoid arthritis examined vegetarian or vegan diets. Some showed that these diets benefit people with rheumatoid arthritis but I am not sure whether other foods have not been found as beneficial or whether there have not been enough scientific studies on diet issues generally. The Arthritis Research website indicates that certain diets may be beneficial for some people (see Chapter 4 for further details). In research investigating the role of supplements, some studies indicate positive results from fish oils (see Chapter 4).

Fighting infections

As far as infections go, I have noticed that sometimes my symptoms are worse if I am fighting an infection. Often the infection does not develop but the rheumatoid arthritis gets worse. I have noticed that many people who have rheumatoid arthritis seldom have colds and flu and similar infections, probably because of the way the immune system reacts. This is because those of us with rheumatoid arthritis have immune systems that are very active. In a normal immune system there would be extra activity if the body was fighting an infection, but with rheumatoid arthritis the immune system reacts more strongly and the reaction is also likely to carry on longer. This probably means that those of us with rheumatoid arthritis are excellent at fighting off infections but may get symptoms of rheumatoid arthritis such as swelling, pain, stiffness and fatigue instead. It should be noted here that some types of medication suppress the immune system and may also reduce this reaction to some degree (see Chapter 3).

Fatigue

Fatigue is a feeling of both physical and mental weariness and it is the second most common symptom of RA. Some people seem to have more of a problem with fatigue than other people do and also some days, weeks or months can feel worse than others and so it is another unpredictable factor of RA like inflammation and pain. There are many factors that influence how much fatigue we experience when we have RA. A study quoted in a recent rheumatology journal found that over 50% of subjects with RA had high levels of fatigue and that these high levels were linked to pain and depression. Before medical treatment 87% of people had significant fatigue but after medical treatment this had reduced to 50% and this was mostly because the levels of pain had reduced.[8]

Constant pain can wear people down if it continues and so it is very important to control pain as much as possible. Continued pain and fatigue combined with lack of exercise and anxiety about the condition mean that depression is more likely. Then a vicious circle occurs as the depression itself increases the feeling of fatigue. Both pain and depression also interfere with sleep and loss of sleep means more tiredness, leading to more feelings of fatigue.

Of course the levels of disease activity and inflammation also contribute to fatigue because when inflammation is active similar chemicals occur that are found when we have colds and flu. This means that people with very active RA can feel unwell and worn out even though other people cannot see any actual symptoms. Of course it's important to take medication to slow up the disease activity but some drugs used to treat RA can also lead to drowsiness or weariness. Anaemia is also a common symptom of RA and may also be a reason for feelings of fatigue. At the same time weakened and wasting muscles can mean that more energy is needed for everyday activity and this can also make people feel that everything is a struggle on a daily basis.

This all sounds very negative but there are many new treatments now for RA and once a medical treatment is found to slow up the active disease then pain levels can improve and it is easier to sleep. At this stage it is then possible to increase exercise and enjoy some work, social and leisure activities so that depression is reduced. Once the pain and depression are reduced the fatigue will become less troublesome. It then becomes important to find a balance of activities and rest that works on a daily basis.

I have been lucky in that fatigue has not been an enormous problem for me; however, there are many times that I have had to force myself out of bed to go to work whilst feeling as if I am wading through treacle. My limbs feel heavy and stiff and everything is such a struggle. Sometimes it can feel such an effort to get my clothes on, get down the stairs and drive my car to work especially on a day when the car windscreen needs scraping too! I do know that it's worth it to get myself going because once I am involved with work or enjoying time with friends or family I am less aware of what's happening with my body and I forget my own problems.

A personal scenario

In looking for triggers the problem is that there are so many variables and it seems to be very difficult to work out any obvious cause that aggravates symptoms. Even if one person manages this it cannot be generalised to anyone else. This lack of predictability means that sufferers end up feeling powerless and also frustrated because of the difficulty of planning ahead.

My rheumatoid arthritis started with severe pain in my hands and feet and I noticed that I could not shake my wrists whilst I was doing PE with children on my teaching practice (I was on a teachers' training course at the time). About a month or two later, when I was working in a park as a gardener, the pain became even more pronounced. All the other staff in the park were men who were very chauvinistic in their attitude. They thought that cleaning the house, looking after children and cooking was the only work that women should do. I had to prove that I was up to the job. This was difficult to do because every day my feet hurt and the strength in my hands was so reduced that even lifting a large teapot in the staff kitchen was difficult. At night times I put my hands under my pillow to try to reduce the pain so that I could sleep. In the day I carried on digging, hoeing, pruning and driving a tractor. I thought it was only a temporary problem and that it would go away. I did not see a doctor until four months had passed.

Looking back, going to college may have been the factor or one of the factors that triggered the rheumatoid arthritis. I had begun to realise that teaching was not really for me and I was dreading the teaching practices. The rheumatoid arthritis was still active when I went into hospital for an unrelated operation during the following December. During the Christmas holidays I decided to leave college, and the stress went away and with it the rheumatoid arthritis. It may have been the rest and the anaesthetic, or the removal of the stress, or a combination of these things. The rheumatoid arthritis did not reoccur for four years.

The next trigger appeared to be connected to the birth of my three daughters as the rheumatoid arthritis returned when each of my children had reached the age of three months. This personal anecdotal evidence is supported by other studies. A review by Hampl and Papa[9] at Arizona State University concluded that the benefits of pregnancy have been known for decades but only recently have lactation and prolactin been indicated as predictors of onset, flare or relapse of arthritis. It is stated that there is an increased risk of rheumatoid arthritis particularly after the first pregnancy in susceptible women. This seems to have been the case for me. Subsequently the relapses and remissions continued every couple of years for unknown reasons.

Over the last 15 years I have had no remissions and the condition just carries on gradually attacking the joints in my hands and feet, and I also have attacks on my shoulders and knees. The disease is very unpredictable in that it can occur in any joint at any time. I have tried to look for triggers and treatments but with limited success. This situation has made me feel powerless at times and I expect many of you can identify with this feeling. I try to take back some control by being positive, adapting my lifestyle, exercising and working, enjoying leisure pursuits and travelling. Generally, I try to get on with life and forget my disabilities. *It is very important to do this so that you feel you have some control over the condition and therefore over your life.*

My initial contacts with an Occupational Therapist put me on the right track for understanding my condition and achieving a good quality of life. In the next chapters I will outline and discuss the ideas that I have learnt as a patient and also during my training and work as a therapist.

Key points

▶ Rheumatoid arthritis is a disease of the autoimmune system.

▶ In rheumatoid arthritis the immune system attacks its own joints, causing pain and inflammation.

▶ Early diagnosis can help prevent joint deformities.

▶ A problem of the condition is its unpredictability: onset triggers can vary from person to person.

2

Pain and Discomfort: The Key Issues

Pain is a personal experience common to all individuals yet unique to each. (Autton)[1]

One of the key issues for anyone who has rheumatoid arthritis is dealing with pain, stiffness and discomfort. Many people with rheumatoid arthritis rank pain as the most important symptom to be treated. According to the Arthritis Research Campaign (ARC),[2] 50% of people with arthritis say that the worst aspect of having arthritis is the pain. One of the ways that rheumatoid arthritis is diagnosed is by taking a history of a patient's symptoms and these usually include pain, discomfort and/or morning stiffness. Along with these symptoms there is sometimes a feeling of malaise, a feeling that everything is too much of a struggle, particularly at the start of the day. It can therefore be difficult to move around, go to work or carry on activities of daily living.

Coping with pain

The dilemma for anyone suffering from rheumatoid arthritis is that it is preferable to have a job or an occupation because it gives you a reason to get out and about in the morning. This in turn means that muscles, joints, ligaments and tendons are used regularly and do not weaken so quickly. It is important to realise that the stiffness and pain often subside to some degree once you start moving unless you have an intense flare-up. In this case it is better to rest for a few days. Exercise is also good for bones, reducing the risk of osteoporosis. Having a variety of roles like teacher, mother or writer gives people satisfaction, whilst having paid employment improves your standard of living and the range of leisure interests, etc. that you can pursue.

The problem is that when pain is intense it is almost impossible to do anything at all. The experience of pain is unique for each one of us and it is impossible for anyone else to know just exactly what the pain feels like for you. It is therefore very upsetting to be told to ignore the pain and get on with things. *Having rheumatoid arthritis means you have to continually balance what you do in your life.*

Medication will reduce pain and inflammation to some degree, but what is the payoff in side effects? It is also true that some drugs mask pain so that the joint is not rested when it needs to be. If there is a flare-up then rest is essential, but what if you cannot rest because there are children to look after or a job to go to? The problem is that it is also important to carry on these roles if you can but the work and rest balance needs to be right. Life becomes meaningless if you cannot do some of the things that you want to do, but it is also important to protect your joints and your energy levels. We all need to find the balance that is right for ourselves. If possible, we need to find a way to reduce the pain and stiffness that we experience.

There is no complete answer to the problem of pain, but understanding it better may give insight into coping with it more successfully. The next section of this chapter outlines why we have pain and then looks briefly at pain reduction techniques. Many of these will be examined in more detail later in the book.

Understanding pain

The word 'pain' is derived from the word *poena*, which means punishment. It is a very unpleasant sensory experience, which occurs because there either is, has been or is likely to be tissue damage. It is difficult to be more specific because the experience is so different for everyone. Clinically pain is often divided into two groups:

- chronic; and
- acute.

Acute pain is relatively short lived. It is usually a warning signal and recedes when action is taken to stop it. We have sensory receptors in our body tissues for heat, pressure or touch and these will respond if the stimulus is strong enough to cause tissue damage. Pain will then be felt, action will be taken and the pain will subside. For instance, this happens when you burn yourself on a pan.

On the other hand, chronic pain is persistent and carries on long after healing is complete. It is unlikely that it can be serving any useful biological function during this time.

There is no clear dividing line between active and chronic pain and, in rheumatoid arthritis, both may occur.

In rheumatoid arthritis acute pain usually occurs because during inflammation the joint capsule or ligament is stretched. Pain could also be due to pressure on blood vessels or compression of a nerve or because there is tension in muscles. The pain may be a warning of internal tissue damage to the cartilage and lining of the joints. In some people with rheumatoid arthritis the pain seems to persist as chronic pain when a flare-up has ended and there should be remission. This may be because, when the tissues were damaged, nerves could have been damaged too and the central nervous system may have been affected. Sensation in the area of damage might have become heightened, producing persistent chronic pain.

The pain gate

Understanding pain mechanisms can help in the reduction of pain. The mechanism for pain is a complex process involving mental and physical components and is called the **pain gate theory**. This theory proposes that there is a neural mechanism that acts like a 'gate'. It is a highly specialised system of cells that receive input from large and small diameter nerve fibres. These fibres come from the sense receptors of the body and from the brain. The opening and closing of the gate depends on the relative activity of the large diameter and small diameter fibres. We have transmission cells called T cells projecting into the brain and it is these that start the production of pain. Activity of the large diameter cells tends to stop the transmission of the T cells and therefore no pain is felt. Activity in the small diameter fibres tends to open the gate and pain occurs. This research has led to more understanding of pain and how it is possible to stimulate the large diameter fibres and close the pain gate. Mechanical or electrical stimulation can stimulate these fibres and so close the pain gate.

The TENS machine

The principle of electrical stimulation is used in the Transcutaneous Electrical Nerve Stimulation (TENS) device and other similar devices that are now on sale. These machines seem to achieve some degree of relief in about 60% of sufferers, although the success with chronic pain is only about 30%. McQuay *et al*[3] summarised their findings about pain relief in 1997. They stated that the TENS machine was beneficial when used in large doses and that its effectiveness increased over time.

Physiotherapy departments usually have TENS machines or similar devices and some retailers offer demonstrations and approval periods with money-back guarantees. The TENS unit is a small box with adhesive pads that go onto your skin. It is always necessary to try equipment before purchase because everyone is an individual and what works for one person will not necessarily work for another.

Massage

Massage produces mechanical stimulation and can therefore also be effective at reducing pain. Many types of massage are available including aromatherapy. This is a type of massage using oils that can be chosen specifically to be beneficial for arthritis. Aromatherapy is wonderfully relaxing, easing tension particularly around the neck area and generally easing pain. I have not found any research specifically indicating the use of massage or aromatherapy for rheumatoid arthritis. However, there is research to show that relaxation is beneficial in reducing pain. I have tried aromatherapy a few times and I have found that it does reduce tension and that it allows my joints to move more easily. The problem is that it is not available on the National Health Service (NHS) and is therefore expensive to have regularly.

You can buy massage equipment from many retail outfits and these can be used with or without oils. You can massage yourself or get a partner to do it for you. Alternatively there are massage courses available and you can attend with a friend or a partner to learn basic massage techniques.

I also find that heat is useful to reduce discomfort. You can buy a hot water bottle or, nowadays, you can buy wheat bags that you put into a microwave to heat up. These are very useful as you do not have to fill them like bottles and you can drape them around your neck or put them over or under your feet or in the curve of your back. They are not very expensive and are well worth bearing in mind for your Christmas or birthday list.

Acupuncture

Acupuncture is also used for pain relief because it, too, produces an intense sensory input. Needles are inserted in specific points of the body to clear energy channels. The needles may close the pain gate or it may be that they stimulate the production of endorphins, the body's natural painkillers. It is difficult to know how effective acupuncture is for rheumatoid arthritis. One study in *Rheumatology* journal in 1999 concluded that acupuncture was not useful for rheumatoid arthritis patients.[4] Another study by Berman *et al* in the USA[5] also concluded that the usefulness of acupuncture for rheumatoid arthritis has not been demonstrated on a large scale. It appears to be more useful for the pain caused by osteoarthritis. It may, however, be worth a try and sometimes it is possible for a GP to make a referral for acupuncture. At present there is a move for complementary treatments and therapies to be funded by the NHS so it may soon be possible to try massage in this way as well.

Distraction

Another way to reduce the impact of pain is to use the idea of distraction. This means that you need to choose an activity that is totally absorbing and enjoyable. This may then distract you from feeling the pain, at least temporarily, or it may reduce the impact of the pain. In my own case I use music: listening, performing, dancing or going to concerts. Music has always been very important to me but it is only recently that I came across a book exploring the healing effects of music, called *The Mozart Effect*.[6]

This book illustrates the benefits of music of all types and shows how different types of music can be appropriate for different conditions and for strengthening the mind. This is how music can be useful for reducing pain. Certainly music can help us to express emotions and it can change our mood. Depending on the type of music, we can feel full of energy, sad, relaxed or happy. Music has always seemed to be beneficial for me but all of us must find an appropriate activity for ourselves. Obviously it must be something that can be realistically managed. It could be a film or an absorbing book or it could be attending a football match or bird watching or socialising. It really does not matter what it is. As long as you enjoy it you will find that it can reduce the sensation of pain for a time.

Natural pain-killers

If the activity you choose is a physical activity then this will also have the added bonus of stimulating endorphins, the natural pain-killers that our own body produces. This type of pain-control mechanism can be seen in cases where people have suffered a serious injury but are somehow able to get to safety and do not feel pain until later. Producing these endorphins is nature's way of ensuring the best chance of survival.

Laughter also seems to work by promoting good circulation and/or by stimulating the release of endorphins. It is therefore very important to have fun, do things that you enjoy and find something to make you laugh. Recent research has shown the benefits of a good laugh. In his book *The Healing Journey*[7] Matthew Manning tells us:

patients who seem to experience the lowest levels of pain are invariably those who can laugh, sometimes at themselves, in times of difficulty or danger.

Nutrition

It may be possible to alter the balance of the chemicals in your body by exploring nutritional changes and supplements. There are many books and articles claiming that certain diets and supplements can cure arthritis pain. However, reading books on food guidelines can be confusing and research is inconclusive. There is no general cure for rheumatoid arthritis that can work for everyone, although some people do seem to derive benefits from avoiding certain foods. This may be because some people have a food allergy that aggravates the rheumatoid arthritis symptoms. This will be discussed further in Chapter 4, 'Complementary Approaches' but for everyone with RA it is definitely a good idea not to put on too much weight if possible because it puts a further strain on the joints and makes pain and damage more likely. A healthy diet which includes all essential vitamins and minerals, particularly calcium, is very important. This is because it is important to keep the bones and joints as strong as possible. Osteoporosis tends to be more common in rheumatoid arthritis patients, probably because of reduced exercise or because of steroid treatments.

Relaxation

Using relaxation techniques, yoga or hydrotherapy can reduce the tension in our bodies. Some techniques are more useful than others. The best type of relaxation for people with rheumatoid arthritis involves the use of visualisation, rather than the sort that involves tightening and releasing muscles. It is also important to remember to notice when your muscles are tensed up, so that you learn to stay as relaxed as possible, because tension creates pain. A study by Affleck *et al*[8] in 1992, carried out on 75 rheumatoid arthritis patients, showed that patients who used relaxation daily had less pain for the duration of the study. Relaxation and stress management will be discussed in more detail in a later chapter.

Posture

It is also important that a correct posture is adopted for sitting, standing and walking. Often we are not aware of the inappropriate ways we do things until it is pointed out. I often used to stand in a way that put all my weight onto the same foot.

Being aware of what to look for means that you become more observant of the positions that you adopt. Bad posture can also increase pain. There will be further discussion of posture in a later chapter and guidelines on correct posture for reducing pain.

Changing positions

Continually changing the position of your joints is also extremely beneficial. It is really necessary to change positions frequently, about every 20 minutes. I find that if I go to the cinema then I have to really struggle to get out of the seat at the end of the film, and also that my shoulders are very stiff and rigid and I cannot put my coat on.

However, if I am in the house, carrying out light domestic tasks, my joints feel much less stiff.

My work environment is also beneficial for me, as in the office all the resources and forms are a long way away so I have to continually get up and down. I also have to go on home visits that involve driving and walking as well as sitting down, so this means that I regularly change my position and the joints that I am using.

The pain diary

Another idea that may be useful for reducing pain is keeping a **pain diary**. Many variables can be recorded, for example food, activity, the weather and stress. These should be recorded one at a time to see if a pattern emerges. The pain should be scored according to intensity from 1 to 5. Make a recording for morning, afternoon, evening and night. The diary should be kept for about a month for each type of variable. It can be helpful to keep a diary even if a pattern does not emerge, because it often shows that the pain or stiffness is not always present to the same degree. If a pattern does emerge then the day can be planned more efficiently.

I always start my day very slowly and take a long time to get up. I have a cup of tea in bed and exercise my joints in bed by gently moving and stretching my shoulders, arms, fingers, legs and toes. I then get up slowly and gradually I loosen up. I drive to work and I am still fairly stiff when I arrive, mostly because of having to sit in the car in traffic. I wander around at work and have a coffee. Three hours after I have woken up I feel a bit more human!

Splinting

If pain is very intense in the hands then splints can be beneficial and an Occupational Therapy department will give out working splints. These reduce pain by ensuring that the painful joint does not move or get knocked when you are doing activities. Many patients find these splints useful. A study in the *Journal of Rheumatology*[9] in 1998 examined the effects of the wrist orthosis (splint) on work performance and pain. Pain was found to be significantly less after work if the splint was worn. Nocturnal resting splints can also be provided by OT departments. These splints are worn at night both to reduce pain and to keep the fingers of the hand in a more extended position to try to prevent deformities. A study in the *American Journal of Occupational Therapy*[10] concluded that resting hand splints are effective for pain relief. However, I have been unable to find research establishing that resting splints reduce deformities in the hands, but this could be because the research has not been done.

Medication

Of course the main way that people control pain is by using medication. Some medication is given to slow down the rate of disease progression and some is given for relief of inflammation and pain control. The medication available for rheumatoid arthritis will be discussed in more detail in the next chapter. Generally, it is important that you as a patient ensure that you understand what a particular medication does and what the likely side effects are. It is essential that all medication is reviewed regularly and that you take blood tests where these are necessary. It is also important to make sure that appointment times with consultants are used as fully as possible. Always think out any questions that you want answered and jot them down so that you do not forget.

There are many pros and cons to taking regular medication and it is always a balancing act. Each individual must decide with the help of his or her consultant rheumatologist. *It is important that you make an informed choice*. The Arthritis Research Campaign website www.arc.org.uk keeps a lot of useful information and this can enable you to make a decision.

Surgery

If pain is persistent, and it is preventing the joint from moving properly and reducing your ability to walk or care for yourself, then surgery may sometimes be suggested. This could be an operation to:

- fuse a joint to make it more stable;
- replace a badly damaged joint with an artificial joint;
- remove the inflamed lining of the joint cavity;
- remove the painful coverings from tendons or repairing damaged tendons;
- remove bone to relieve pain;

■ release trapped nerves.

If the joint is fused it will stop the pain but obviously the joint movement will be lost. A replacement may be suggested but this will depend on the damage done, the pain and how much it affects daily activities. It will also depend on your age and lifestyle because some replacements may not last more than ten or 15 years and will have to be updated regularly. However joint replacements are being improved all the time and some replacement joints can last more than 20 years. You will need to weigh up the pros and cons and discuss the operation with your consultant. It is not advisable to rush into surgery but it could be very beneficial.

The most common joint replacements are knuckles (MCP joints), hips and knees. The knuckle joints have been improving and now may be recommended if you have deformities and/or pain in the fingers. The artificial replacement joints can correct the alignment of the fingers, reduce pain and allow more normal hand function. If you have damage to the middle finger joints as well then the result will not be as good but may still bring about improvements. A lot of exercise is needed after the operation to stretch the tendons and strengthen the muscles and you will need to work hard at this in order to achieve the desired results.

Many of the other most widely performed operations are carried out to improve hand function and/or reduce pain in the fingers and wrist. I am not going to go into the details of all these operations here because the Arthritis Research website has very good information on these operations. However, I have included a brief summary of the most common operations for the hand and wrist.

Wrist fusion

This surgery may be suggested if the wrist joint is badly damaged and causing a lot of pain. The operation usually eliminates pain and increases strength; however, it's important to bear in mind that there will be no wrist movement afterwards. It will still be possible to manage most tasks by finding different ways to do them but with no wrist movement the fingers will gradually start to deviate to compensate. I have not had any wrist movement since my late twenties as the wrists fused by themselves. The only things that come to mind that are difficult or impossible for me are pushing myself up from the ground or from a bath, cleaning windows, playing badminton and sports that require wrist movement, opening child-proof medication bottles and doing press-ups. It is also a bit harder to use keyboards. **Thumb joint fusion** may also be offered if there is extensive pain in the middle joint.

Carpal tunnel syndrome release

Carpal tunnel syndrome occurs when there is pressure on the median nerve as it passes through the wrist. This produces a lot of pain in the wrist. Surgery is sometimes needed to relieve the pressure on the nerve and therefore stop the pain. The operation is done by dividing the carpal tunnel ligament that passes over the nerve. Exercising the fingers after the operation is very important in order to prevent the nerve and the tendons becoming caught up in the scar tissue. The exercise also prevents the joints becoming stiff.

Trigger finger release

Sometimes the tendon in a finger joint makes it difficult for a finger to move correctly and the result is that every now and then it will get stuck and then suddenly it will work, causing a trigger movement. An operation is sometimes needed to release the tendon.

Tendon transfers or repairs

Tendons in the hand can occasionally rupture. This causes problems either with bending or straightening the fingers, depending on whether the flexor or extensor tendons are affected. The tendon will be repaired if it's caught early enough but otherwise a good tendon will need to be transferred from another finger. After the initial splinting period a long period of exercise will be needed to get the tendon working successfully.

Unfortunately the surgery may not be performed at the time when it is most beneficial because of waiting times to see the consultant and to have the operation. This happened to me when I needed a tendon operation. Anyone waiting for surgery can find that tendons have shortened and then the joints cannot work properly even when the surgery has been performed. Also, waiting often puts the strain onto other joints and then they may well become damaged and painful too. If it is an option it is a good idea to pay privately, at least for the consultation. Also a second opinion may be a good idea.

A personal scenario

I have had rheumatoid arthritis for 30 years and luckily for me the only time I had extensive and continuous pain was in the early years before diagnosis. At this time my hands and feet were painful most of the time, and at night it was intensive and I found it difficult to sleep. Since then I have experienced a lot of stiffness and discomfort but the only time I have had intense pain is when someone has tried to force a joint into a position that has become almost impossible due to joint damage. For instance, when my children were small they moved quickly and unexpectedly, and knocked my hands or sat on my feet before I could jump out of the way. At other times I might knock into things or I might get a recoil reaction from pushing or pulling something. This pain is intense but it is short-lived and is therefore bearable. A quick scream makes you feel better!

I am not sure whether I control pain by my lifestyle, by exercising, practising joint protection techniques, keeping active, relaxing or by taking medication, or whether it is my chemical and biological make-up that helps by producing lots of endorphins. It may well be all of these things. I only know that I do not seem to suffer the pain that many people do. I consequently seem to be a bit of an enigma to many of my doctors and therapists. In the rest of this book I will discuss these issues in more depth in the hope that I can help others to have a good quality of life and freedom from pain.

Key points

- ▶ Acute and chronic pain, stiffness and discomfort are often key issues for people with rheumatoid arthritis.
- ▶ Understanding pain mechanisms can help reduce pain.
- ▶ You can reduce pain through a variety of methods such as relaxation, medication, massage, acupuncture, TENS machine, nutrition, splinting, posture, etc.
- ▶ Keeping a pain diary can help you to see patterns and to plan your day.

3

Understanding Medication

Knowledge is power.

If you have rheumatoid arthritis it is useful to be aware of the main types of medication used in controlling rheumatoid arthritis and its symptoms. You should have a general understanding of how the different medications work and what they should achieve. You will probably need to read information leaflets because often it can be difficult to ask all the questions that you need to when you have an appointment with a consultant. This is mainly because of time constraints, but it is also because we as patients tend to worry that a question is pointless or inappropriate, or sometimes we just forget because there is often a long wait to be seen by the consultant. This has certainly happened to me, especially when I had to wait regularly over an hour with three small children. I had to remember to write questions out and take them in with me.

We need to know:

- what medication we are taking;
- how to take it; and
- why it is necessary.

The choice of medication should be discussed and we should be actively involved in decisions concerning medication. We need to be informed so that we can make an appropriate choice. Anyone who is taking medication for long-term use should be aware of possible side effects and the need for monitoring their condition.

As patients we need to take a share of the responsibility for managing our condition, but it is vital that we have information before we can take an active role. Ask for information leaflets, check the arthritis websites (see Useful Resources) and make a list of questions to ask when you see your consultant. Anyone who is not happy with the relationship that they have with their consultant is entitled to ask their doctor to refer them for a second opinion. In fact this may be useful anyway as all consultants have different opinions and it is often useful to listen to a different point of view. A lot of people are reluctant to do this for fear that it will jeopardise their relationship with their existing consultant. There are some grounds for this and asking to see another consultant should be done tactfully via the GP.

There are so many medications available now for rheumatoid arthritis that it can be quite confusing understanding which drugs do what and why you are taking them. I will therefore outline the types of medication used for rheumatoid arthritis. This is only a basic guide and if a more detailed account is needed there are many books available as well as Arthritis Research Campaign leaflets.

Six main types of drugs are used to treat rheumatoid arthritis. These are as follows.

1   **Analgesics.**
2   **Non-steroidal anti-inflammatory drugs** known as **NSAIDs.**
3   **Disease-modifying anti-rheumatic drugs** known as **DMARDs.**
4   **Biological therapies.**
5   **New biological therapies.**
6   **Corticosteroids.**

Drugs have two names: the chemical ingredient name and the manufacturer's 'trade' name – which can be confusing. I have therefore put the trade names in brackets.

1 Analgesics

These are primarily painkillers of various descriptions and do not need to be taken regularly but only when pain needs controlling. You should never take more than the recommended dose as they can be very damaging to internal organs, but the most common side effect is constipation. There are different classes of analgesics and some people may be able to tolerate one class but not another. The problem is that some analgesics are combinations of different classes.

You need to be aware of this if a certain type causes you side effects or is dangerous for you. For instance, paracetamol and codeine are often used in combined preparations and one may be tolerated but not the other. Many painkillers become less effective if used continually. It is better to control pain in other ways if possible. However, it is almost impossible to concentrate on anything else if pain is very intense and in this case there may seem little option.

This group includes: paracetamol, co-codamol, co-dydramol, until recently co-proxamol and di-hydrocodeine.

2 Non-steroidal anti-inflammatory drugs (NSAIDs)

This group works by controlling the prostaglandins that cause inflammation. They therefore reduce inflammation and the subsequent swelling and stiffness. Anyone with rheumatoid arthritis is likely to use these at some time. In mild disease they may be used on their own or with analgesics, or they may be used in conjunction with one or both of the next two groups as well as analgesics if the disease is more serious. These drugs work quickly, within an hour or two, and may last for up to eight or 12 hours or more if they are a slow-release type. They need to be taken for at least five days to achieve the full anti-inflammatory effect. You should always take them with or after food so that the stomach is lined because of the potential side effect of stomach problems. They may also harm the kidneys or increase asthma.

This group includes ibuprofen (Brufen, Nurofen), diclofenac (Voltarol, Diclomax), idometacin (Indocid), naproxen (Naprosyn), piroxicam (Feldene), and nabumetone (Relifex).

There are now some new NSAIDs that should be kinder to the stomach. The older type of NSAIDs inhibit both cox-1 and cox-2 enzymes but cox-1 enzymes are beneficial in protecting the stomach. The new NSAIDs, however, are selective inhibitors of the cox-2 enzyme and so they should give fewer side effects, as there is still some cox-1 enzyme activity. New drugs are being developed in this group with further improvements in side effect profiles, but they all have the same strength and efficacy as other NSAIDs.

This new group of NSAIDs, the coxibs, consists of celecoxib (Celebrex) and etonicoxib (Arcoxia) and two partially selective cox-2 inhibitors meloxicam (Mobic) and Etodolac (Lodine).

3 Disease-modifying anti-rheumatic drugs (DMARDs)

This group of drugs is used by anyone with more serious disease. People with indications of joint damage or extensive inflammation and stiffness will be advised to take them to control the rate of disease and limit damage to the joints. In fact, many people are started on these drugs at an early stage nowadays, because there is a tendency to use aggressive treatment early on in order to try to prevent joint damage. They are slower to become effective and a step-up dose is needed. This means a small dose is taken first then the dosage is gradually increased. It therefore takes up to three months for this type of medication to be fully effective. The medication does not provide a complete cure but only helps to slow down the disease as long as the medication is being taken. The disease is therefore likely to return if the medication is stopped. According to Mason and Smith[1] in their book *Rheumatoid Arthritis: Your Medication Explained* it is common for DMARDs to work for only three to four years. It is also true that some types work for some patients and not for others.

Drugs in this group are immuno-suppressants, meaning that they suppress the immune response. This in turn means that the rate that the joints are attacked and destroyed by the immune system is slowed down. These drugs need to be strong in order to work in this way and therefore you should always ensure that you are being monitored by regular blood tests. You should report any side effects. You should also be aware that some of the drugs in this group may affect fertility and this should be discussed with your consultant if you are intending to start a family. Some drugs may lower the sperm count, e.g. sulphasalazine, azathioprine and methotrexate. Some may affect the ova or cause miscarriages or birth defects, e.g. methotrexate and leflunomide, and some may cause sterility. (See the *Pregnancy and Arthritis* booklet published by ARC for further information.[2]) The medication may need to be stopped three months prior to conceiving.

Examples of this group are: methotrexate, sulphasalazine, lefluno-mide, gold, hydroxychloroquine and azathioprine. Sometimes two of these drugs are combined, e.g. methotrexate and sulphasalazine.

4 Biological therapies

There are also new drugs in this group. These are the anti-TNF drugs also known as the biological therapies. These new drugs work in a different way. People with rheumatoid arthritis have excessive amounts of a protein called TNF and this increases inflammation. These drugs block the TNF and therefore reduce inflammation. They will only be prescribed if other drugs in this group have been tried and have failed and if the disease is very active. The **DAS scoring system** is now often used to establish if someone qualifies for the new biological drugs.

DAS stands for 'disease activity score'. It is a number that measures the activity of the RA. The doctor or nurse calculates the DAS based on several tests. These include the number of tender and swollen joints, an assessment of how the patient feels their condition is affecting them at that time and the results of the most recent blood test. The blood test will show the amount of inflammation present and the activity of the disease. The scoring is interpreted as follows.

- Less than 2.6 Disease remission.
- 2.6 to 3.2 Low disease activity.
- More than 3.2 May merit change in therapy for some patients.
- More than 5.1 Severe disease activity.

Before being considered for the new biological therapies you will need to score at least 3.2 on the DAS. Normally you will also have had to try and fail at least two non biologic DMARDs as well to be con-sidered. This is because they are more expensive than the conventional DMARDs and although there is now more information and evalua-tion of their short term side effects the long-term side effects of these drugs are not known and therefore care should be taken, especially if you want to start a family. This group of drugs is given by injection rather than being taken in tablet form. The infusion may be given in hospital or sometimes it can be given by self-injection. These drugs are often given in conjunction with methotrexate but may be given on their own. According to research concerning early active RA, combinations of DMARDs and TNF/methotrexate combinations are more effective than methotrexate alone. A recent study on combination therapies concludes that there is 'strong evidence in favour of combination treatment for RA but there is still uncertainty about which regimen is preferable.'[3]

The present anti-TNF drugs that are registered for use in the UK are infliximab (Remicade) etanercept (Enbrel) adulimumab (Humira) Golimumab (Simponi) and certolizumab pegol (Cimzia).

5 New biological therapies

There are also some other biological therapies than are not anti-TNF drugs and these have become available recently. They target different processes in the immune system and work in different ways to the first wave of biologics. Arthritis Care states on their website that 20–30% of people with RA do not respond to anti-TNF treatments. There are three other biologicals that may be used in this case. These are as follows.

Rituximab (Mab Thera) is a drug that attacks B-cells and destroys them. B-cells are antibody-producing white blood cells. In the healthy body B-cells are useful for producing antibodies to fight germs but in people with rheumatoid arthritis the B-cells may produce 'autoantibodies' that are very destructive for the joints of people with RA. Research has shown that when the B-cells of patients in a study were destroyed many of those patients showed improvements in their rheumatoid arthritis that were sustained for some months. Rituximab is given by intravenous infusion in hospital. Usually two infusions are given two weeks apart. Many people have rituximab about once a year.

Abatacept (Orencia) is a new drug for RA that was approved by the European Commission in 2010. Abatacept works by blocking the activity of T-cells, which are a type of white blood cell. It makes them inactive and stops a chain of events linked to the immune system targeting the joints. Abatacept is used to treat severe active rheumatoid arthritis, usually in combination with methotrexate. It is available throughout the UK except for Scotland.

Abatacept is administered at hospital through an intravenous infusion (drip) and needs to be monitored closely. The administration takes about 30 minutes every four weeks.

Tocilizumab (RoActemra) works by blocking the interleukin-6 receptor (IL-6R). In people with rheumatoid arthritis a protein called IL-6 is overproduced in the body, causing inflammation and damage to bones, cartilage and tissue. Tocilizumab blocks the action of IL-6 and so can reduce this inflammation and damage. RoActemra (tocilizumab) was launched in the UK in October 2009 and 'new information shows that when it is used with methotrexate, it inhibits progression of joint damage in 83% of people with RA after two years, compared to just 66% of people treated with methotrexate and a placebo.'[4]

Tocilizumab is given by intravenous infusion (a drip) once every four weeks. Each treatment will take about an hour.

6 Corticosteroids (steroids)

These are given in tablet form or as injections. They are disease-modifying drugs as well as powerful anti-inflammatory drugs and they have a very fast response. All in all they sound amazing, but of course such powerful drugs are likely to have serious side effects and, if you are taking them, you should make sure that you are well aware of these. There are both short- and long-term effects from steroid use and it is not unusual to find that people are not aware of these dangers. It is essential to understand all the implications of using them at the outset. If used for a long time (months) or at high doses they produce side effects. Also it is important to note that the body usually has its own supply of this chemical (cortisol) for controlling inflammatory responses in the body. If large doses are taken orally or by injection the body stops producing its own and this is why steroids should never be stopped instantly. They must be gradually reduced so that the body has time to restart its own production.

Another important factor is that steroids are so effective at suppressing the immune response, and therefore preventing the joints from being attacked, that they also make people more vulnerable to other infections and diseases. The steroid used to treat rheumatoid arthritis is prednisolone (Deltacotril, Precortisyl, Predsol).

New treatments

Research is always being carried out to find new treatments. These are often reported in newspapers and on the news and more recently on the internet. It must be remembered that new treatments have to undergo rigorous testing before being made available so nothing happens quickly. It is always a risk to take a new treatment because the long-term side effects will never be known unless the drug has been used for a long time for another condition. It is always necessary to bear this in mind and to weigh up the risks and benefits fully before agreeing to new treatments. However, the outcome of treatment for patients with rheumatoid arthritis has improved considerably during the past 20 years. Several approaches have been investigated, including step-up (adding one drug to another) and step-down (starting with a combination of drugs and withdrawing individual ones) regimens and giving three disease-modifying drugs at the same time. All approaches have reduced inflammatory activity, delayed radiographic progression, and improved function and quality of life although only a few patients have achieved remission.

The future for people with RA has never been brighter however it is still important to recognise that taking medication for a long time means that the liver and kidneys will have extra to cope with. It is therefore a good idea to eat well and not take a lot of alcohol while you are taking medication regularly.

Obviously medication can be very effective in controlling rheumatoid arthritis, but in order to achieve the best possible outcome *it is necessary to make adjustments and changes in many areas of life, and to make use of different treatments and therapies.* The next chapters outline the many ways that you can help yourself to achieve optimum health and wellbeing, even though you have rheumatoid arthritis.

A personal scenario

As far as my personal situation goes I have never been very happy taking medication long-term, although I do recognise that there is a need to control the disease if joints are becoming damaged. *It is a question of balancing the potential benefits against the potential harm.*

In 1974, when I first had intense symptoms of rheumatoid arthritis but no diagnosis, I believe that my doctor felt there may have been psychological harm in telling me that I had rheumatoid arthritis when I was only 22. There may be some justification in this, but the damage to my joints was probably increased because I was not given any disease-modifying drugs and I was not referred to Occupational Therapy to learn about joint protection until I had had rheumatoid arthritis for nearly ten years. I carried on doing potentially damaging actions like lifting heavy prams, pushchairs and babies! Nowadays, people are given disease-modifying medication early on. This probably slows up the disease process and limits the joint damage although it does not cure the rheumatoid arthritis. Hopefully some consultants will also make a referral to Occupational Therapy as well as recommending medication so that patients can achieve the best quality of life and become an expert in managing their own condition.

Key points

▶ Knowing about the main types of medication will help you be involved in what is best for you.

▶ Be aware of any side effects from long-term use of medication.

▶ Six types of drugs are used for rheumatoid arthritis: analgesics, non-steroidal anti-inflammatory drugs, disease-modifying anti-rheumatic drugs, biological therapies, new biological therapies and steroids.

▶ Be prepared to try different treatments and therapies and to make changes in many areas of your life.

4

Complementary Approaches

Food for thought.

Over the last few years there has been more and more interest in complementary therapies. When I first wrote this book there had been little research in this area and therefore evidence was very thin on the ground. There is still a long way to go but a lot of research has now been carried out by Arthritis Research UK (formerly the Arthritis Research Campaign) and other arthritis support organisations. I am grateful to them for the research they have undertaken to clarify the findings of other studies.

The first part of this chapter is an overview of the supplements and foods that are thought to be beneficial for people with RA. There is then some information about healthy diets and food allergies and after this I have included information on some of the other complementary therapies that appear to be working for some people either in reducing pain or inflammation.

Beneficial foods and food supplements

Olive oil

A study was carried out by the medical school in Athens University comparing Greek and British patients who had RA. It was found that the severity of the disease was significantly lower among the Greek rheumatoid arthritis patients.[1] Greek people traditionally eat more fruit, vegetables, fish and olive oil than British people and this is perhaps the reason that their disease is not as severe. During many periods of the year the traditional Greek people have also given up meat and meat products for religious reasons and this may also be another reason that their health is better.

This type of Mediterranean diet has been found in studies to give positive benefits to people with RA, reducing inflammation and stiffness and improving strength. One reason for this may be that olive oil contains oleic acid, a monosaturated fatty acid that is converted to molecules with a much lower inflammatory potential. British people tend to eat less olive oil and more animal fats or vegetable oils obtained from sunflower oil or corn oil and these contain more omega 6 fatty acids that participate in inflammation. The oily fish that the Greeks eat also helps to reduce inflammation.

Fish oils

The most commonly used supplement for arthritis is probably fish oil and cod liver oil and some studies of cod liver oil have indicated positive results for people with RA. Volker *et al*[2] carried out research on 50 subjects with RA over a 15-week period. The subjects' clinical status improved. Harwood and Caterson[3] discovered that the omega 3 fatty acids in cod liver oil switch off the enzymes that break down joint cartilage; therefore taking this supplement can reduce cartilage destruction and so reduce pain and stiffness. Fish oils are dietary supplements that are rich in omega-3 essential fatty acids. These fatty acids have strong anti-inflammatory properties because they reduce the release of pro-inflammatory elements from the white blood cells and help in the production of anti-inflammatory substances in the blood (prostaglandins). They also provide vitamin A, which is an antioxidant that can help prevent cell damage in the body as well as providing vitamin D, which helps in maintaining a healthy musculoskeletal system including the cartilage.

You can buy supplements from health food shops or mail order as well as online. The capsules are usually 1 g (1,000 mg) but they are not the pure essential fatty acids DHA and EPA. This means that even with 'high strength' preparations you may need four to five capsules per day. You need to be prepared to take them for at least three months to find out if they are helping you.

I used to be confused between cod liver oil and fish oil in the past and it is important not to confuse them. They both contain omega-3 polyunsaturated fatty acids as well as vitamin D but it is dangerous to take fish liver oils, like cod liver oil, in the large doses recommended for arthritis because of the risk of overdosing with vitamin A.

This is particularly important for pregnant women, or women who might become pregnant, because too much vitamin A can harm the unborn baby.

Borage seed oil

This supplement is derived from the plant seed oil. Borage seed oil is rich in essential fatty acids that can help to regulate the immune system of the body and fight joint inflammation. Present evidence suggests that borage seed oil may improve rheumatoid arthritis disease-related symptoms. The Arthritis Research website quotes two randomised controlled trials that both found a significant difference in the treatment outcomes of the two patient groups in favour of borage seed oil. In one of these trials, after six months of treatment, 'an improvement in joint tenderness and morning stiffness was achieved by 64% of patients on borage seed oil compared to only 21% in those who were on the placebo treatment'.[4]

Capsules are available in doses from 500 mg to 1,300 mg. The capsule usually contains 23% of essential fatty acid GLA. It is not yet clear what an effective dose would be for people with arthritis.

Glucosamine sulphate

This is another supplement that has become popular lately but I could not find any evidence indicating its beneficial effects for RA, although studies on supplements and complementary treatments have not been conducted until recently. I have included it because one study I looked at showed benefits for osteoarthritis (OA) and many people with RA tend to develop OA later on in life. The *Arthritis Bible* also summarises seven controlled trials with positive results, but again these are all for OA.[5]

CMO

In the 1970s a US research scientist called Harry Diehl discovered that he and other researchers could not induce arthritis in mice. He wanted to know what was protecting them and found out that they contained cetyl myristoleate (CMO), a previously unknown fatty acid. He tried to interest pharmaceutical companies in his discovery but was unable to. He did however launch CMO as a dietary supplement in 1991. A trial by Siemandi in 1997 gave very positive results for CMO.[6] According to Dr Len Sands[7] this supplement regulates the immune system and therefore does not need to be taken after the initial few weeks. This is lucky because it is extremely expensive. More research needs to be done on this product to verify the impressive claims that are made. The *Arthritis Bible* gives information on this supplement and others. It is a comprehensive guide to conventional and alternative treatments for arthritis and a very useful book on this subject.

Ginger (Zingiber officinale)

Ginger contains active ingredients that may have analgesic and anti-inflammatory properties and it is shown to increase circulation in people with Raynaud's phenomenon. Studies have shown that ginger extract inhibited inflammation-causing chemicals, including TNF-α and COX-2.[8] Ginger can interfere with medications for blood thinning and should not be used if you have gallstones. Like all supplements, it's advisable to check with your GP before starting supplements if you are taking conventional medications. Ginger can be taken as powder, extract, tincture, capsules or oils.

SKI 306X

SKI 306X is a mixture of three herbs The arthritis research website states that 'Laboratory and animal studies have found that SKI 306X prevents the destruction of proteoglycan and collagen that are important components of joint cartilage' and that. 'Other studies have shown that it can prevent the release of inflammatory substances in joints.' It goes on to say that 'One trial in rheumatoid arthritis showed SKI 306X to be as effective as the NSAID celecoxib.'[9]

SKI 306X tablets are made in 200 mg tablets can can be purchased online. The suggested dosage is 600 mg per day in three separate doses.

Nutrition

As well as using supplements it may be possible to alter the balance of the chemicals in your body by exploring nutritional changes. There are many books and articles claiming that certain diets and supplements can cure arthritis pain. However, reading books on food guidelines can be confusing and research is inconclusive. Some studies have demonstrated that a vegetarian or vegan diet is beneficial, for instance, McDougall et al[10] concluded that 'patients with moderate to severe RA who switch to a low fat vegan diet can experience significant reductions in RA symptoms'. A controlled trial by Kjeldsen-Kragh et al also advocated a vegetarian diet.[11] They reported that RA patients could improve by fasting and then changing to a vegetarian diet.

A study by Palmblad et al in 1991[12] claimed that 'total fasting induces within a few days a substantial reduction of joint swelling, morning stiffness and other arthritic symptoms.' Buchanan et al[13] claim that symptoms are probably reduced in this case because after fasting there are less of the chemicals needed to start the inflammation process. Therefore the reason for the reduction of symptoms could be because of this and not because of a food allergy. Obviously fasting cannot be used as pain relief but only as a way of cleansing the body prior to a diet change. Arthritis Research UK concludes that there is some scientific evidence that the right diet may help symptoms in some people.[14] Whatever diet you try, ensure that you do not leave out essential nutrients.

Fruit and vegetables

The World Health Organisation recommends five portions of fruit and vegetables every day. This is to make sure our body receives the important nutrients it needs like vitamins, minerals and antioxidants. For people with arthritis this is even more important because antioxidants help to protect joints by 'mopping up' some of the body chemicals that cause inflammation. Arthritis Research UK states that research has shown that people who eat plenty of fresh fruit and vegetables, especially the ones containing vitamin C, seem to have a lower risk of developing inflammatory arthritis. Brightly coloured vegetable and fruits are richer in antioxidants.

Calcium

A healthy diet, including all essential vitamins and minerals, particularly calcium, is very important. This is because people with RA need to keep the bones and joints as strong as possible and also osteoporosis tends to be more common in people with RA, probably because of reduced exercise or because of steroid treatments. The richest sources of calcium are milk, cheese, yoghurt, fish with the bones and calcium-enriched soya milk. Unfortunately many people who are trying to lose weight tend to cut out dairy produce and osteoporosis is becoming more common even among the general population. It should also be noted that skimmed or semi-skimmed milk contains more calcium than full-fat milk so if weight is a problem then this is the answer.

Vitamin D
Vitamin D is also needed so that the body is able to absorb the calcium and there is some evidence that arthritis progresses faster in people who are low in it. The body produces vitamin D when we are outside in the sun, so a slight deficiency is quite common in winter but again some people are so worried about skin cancer that they do not get enough regular sunlight. Half an hour a day has been recommended more recently. Vitamin D can be obtained from the diet especially from oily fish or from supplements.

Iron
Many people with rheumatoid arthritis are anaemic and therefore need more iron. However, the anaemia can be due to different causes and is not always related to a shortage of iron. NSAIDs may cause bleeding and stomach ulcers in some people and this can lead to anaemia. There are also some people with RA who are anaemic but are not able to absorb the iron even if they eat iron-rich foods. If this is the case the deficiency should be picked up in blood tests and then it will need more investigation.

Iron is found in red meat, oily fish like sardines, pulses like lentils and haricot beans and dark green vegetables, especially spinach, kale and watercress. It may be best to avoid drinking tea with your meal as it may reduce the amount of iron that your body can absorb.

Selenium
I once visited a homeopath many years ago and he told me to ensure I had selenium in my diet. Consequently I have always eaten lots of

brazil nuts which are a very good source of selenium although there is also some selenium in meat and fish and it can be bought as a supplement. Selenium may be helpful for RA but the reason is not really clear. Some studies have found that people with rheumatoid arthritis have low levels of selenium in their blood compared with people who don't have the disease so this may be significant but it is not known why this is happens or how it may help to alleviate RA. I carried on eating brazil nuts anyway as incidentally they helped with menopause symptoms.

Other dietary considerations

Risk of food-borne infections

People on biological therapy and/or methotrexate should be aware of the risk of food-borne infections due to fact that these drugs suppress the immune system. It is therefore more important to take care with food. Listeria is commonly found in unpasteurised dairy products such as milk and soft cheese plus processed meats, hot dogs and refrigerated pâté. Salmonella may be found in raw or partially cooked egg, poultry and meat. Food should be cooked thoroughly and all leftovers stored in the fridge to stop food-poisoning bacteria growing.

Food Allergies

There is no diet for RA that can help everyone although research has shown that some people can have an improvement in their symptoms by excluding some foods, although the reasons for this aren't yet clear. It may be because some people have a food allergy that aggravates the RA symptoms. Arthritis Research UK says that NSAIDs increase the permeability of the gut and this allows larger molecules of food to pass through than would normally be the case, causing food sensitivity.

Food allergies occur when our immune system mistakenly believes that something we have eaten is harmful. Trying to protect us, the immune system produces immunoglobulin E, also called IgE antibodies, against that food. The antibodies set off a chain reaction that causes symptoms. In some people, the antibodies and proteins bind together and form immune complexes in the intestine. These immune complexes then circulate and may contribute to inflammation, Once antibodies are made against a particular food, the body instantly recognises that food the next time it is eaten and the cycle begins again, causing the symptoms to recur.

Researchers at the University of Oslo, Norway, found that the intestinal fluid of people with RA had higher levels of antibodies to proteins from cow's milk, cereal, hen's eggs, codfish and pork than that of people without RA.[15] Although the proteins were added in a test tube to the subject's intestinal fluids, the people had not actually eaten the foods, so it is not conclusive.

It is probably worthwhile exploring nutrition to find out which foods could make the inflammation worse. Nutritional consultants can do an assessment and then give guidelines as to which foods to avoid and which to eat more of. The guidelines are based on a holistic look at the health problems encountered on an individual basis. The treatment is therefore specific to each person. Alternatively you could try an elimination diet, which involves living on water and herbal teas for two days and then introducing different food types gradually every couple of weeks. Keep a food diary to record food and pain levels. It may then be possible to see if any foods affect you adversely. It could work for you. It didn't work for me, thankfully. I love my food too much!

Reducing weight

It is definitely a good idea not to put on too much weight if possible because it puts a further strain on the joints and makes pain and damage more likely. It is therefore important to reduce fat intake, but remember that calcium is important so do not reduce the fats completely. It's all about balance. Fats are very confusing but basically there are three kinds of fats in foods.

Saturates are mostly of animal origin and found in full-fat dairy products, processed foods like biscuits, cakes and pastry, chips (if fried in animal fat) and Asian foods, especially meals cooked using ghee (clarified butter). There are also some vegetable oils such as palm oil and coconut oil that contain a lot of saturates. Saturated fats are the most important kind of fat to reduce since it is thought that they may increase the pain and inflammation in the body as well as increasing weight.

Monounsaturates are found in olive and rapeseed oil. These are 'neutral' fats in that they do not worsen inflammation, but they contain just as many calories as saturated fats, so it's still important to reduce them if you're trying to lose weight.

Polyunsaturates are softer fats and oils that come from corn or sunflower sources and they are high in omega-6 polyunsaturates. Lately it has been shown that these can increase general inflammation in the body.

In order to reduce and maintain a healthy weight it is also important not to eat too many carbohydrates. People who do not exercise a lot do not need to eat as much food as those people who are generally active. It is also true that as we get older we do not need as much food as when we were younger so although eating is very enjoyable we need to find a balance of activity and food intake that works to maintain a healthy weight and then stick to it. I find the best way to 'diet' is to listen to my body and only eat when I'm hungry rather than nibbling a lot. I have to eat a lot less now than I used to when I was young and energetic. This plan generally works for me except at Christmas when there are far too many chocolate sweets around!

Food is a very complicated subject but I hope this information has given some food for thought. I would now like to consider some of the complementary therapies that certainly appear to be useful for some people in alleviating symptoms like stiffness and pain as well as promoting better health and well-being.

Complementary therapies

Hypnosis

Hypnosis is a deeply relaxed state, induced by a practitioner. You are given therapeutic suggestions to encourage changes in your thinking and behaviour and these changes may lead to the relief of your symptoms. For instance, the suggestion may be given that the joints are improving each day or that your health is getting better each day or that you are turning down the pain each day like the volume of a radio. The suggestions may be recorded so that you can play them back at least daily to implant them in your subconscious mind. The Arthritis Research website states that 'there is scientific evidence that hypnosis can improve pain, physical and psychosocial function in people with arthritis'.[16]

I have experienced hypnotherapy on a number of occasions and it was certainly very good for deep relaxation and I can now relax myself very well and this is useful to recharge energy levels. I personally did not gain any improvement in the symptoms of RA; however, it's difficult to persist in playing the recordings for a long enough period of time for at least two or three times a day consistently in order to really test it out. The sessions are also expensive, as are all complementary therapies, although there are some GPs who also practise hypnotherapy so it may be possible to have it paid for by the NHS.

Magnet therapy

Magnet therapy involves placing magnets or magnetic devices on or near the skin to relieve pain. Magnets can be used in different ways, including jewellery and various magnetic devices, including mattress pads, massage equipment and shoe inserts. The Arthritis Research Organisation states that 'One of the biggest surprises thrown up by recent research is the finding that magnets can be helpful for pain, including low back and knee pain'[17] and ehow.com[18] gives the following information. In an American study 64 patients over the age of 18 years with rheumatoid arthritis and persistent knee pain were investigated. After wearing magnets for one week, 68% of the treatment group (patients who received working magnets) reported feeling better or much better, compared with 27% of the control group (patients who received sham magnets).

It is difficult to know which magnetic system works best but according to your lifestyle a consultant for magnet therapy can help you make suitable choices. It is safe so it definitely may be worth a try.

Homeopathy

This is a very traditional system of medicine that is based on treating like with like. Therefore in an inflammatory disease the treatment would be something to induce inflammation and then the body should respond by producing its own cure. Homeopathic remedies are available over the counter but you should see a practitioner if you are interested because treatments are individual and there is no such thing as a cure for arthritis. The cure is specific to the individual being prescribed for. According to the Arthritis Research UK website a number of carefully controlled trials have been carried out and the results have been inconsistent for rheumatoid arthritis. Homeopathy is available on the NHS as some GPs are also qualified in homeopathy as well as more conventional medical treatments.

Herbalism

Herbalism is said to work by stimulating the natural healing processes of the body so that it can be rebalanced and cleansed. It is interesting that many of the drugs we now use were developed by isolating the key active ingredient from a plant and then synthesising a new drug based on that ingredient. Herbalists say that plants actually work better as they have the key ingredient and others too and this gives a better overall effect. Herbs have antibacterial and antiviral properties and may therefore have a part to play in improving our health. Practitioners believe that if they are correctly prescribed, herbs can be combined and targeted to activate, regulate and heal any organ in the body unless the tissue has been completely destroyed.

The Arthritis Research website has been researching many of these herbal remedies but there is not yet enough research to be able to recommend any particular plants as generally beneficial except perhaps devil's claw (made from a plant that grows in Namibia), Boswellia (from the frankincense tree) and rosehip. Herbalists will recommend a mixture of plant extracts according to symptoms because what works for one person is often not effective for another person. There is no general cure for RA and this is the case for most complementary therapies and indeed for any type of medication.

A personal scenario

I have tried out many complementary treatments over the years but it has always been difficult to work out how beneficial the treatments have actually been. There are a number of reasons for this. RA is very variable and can go into remission and then start up again months or years later. Even in an active period of the disease it can vary on a daily basis so it's difficult to judge what's helping.

Any scientist will tell you that in order to test the effects of a treatment or therapy only one thing at a time should change and everything else should remain the same. This means that your diet, exercise, levels of stress, exposure to infections, relationships, RA medication and everything else in your life needs to remain constant during the period of testing – and this of course is impossible! Our lives are not that simple.

The best approach is to take one new treatment at a time for at least three months, try not to change anything else in your life and see what happens. Then carry on with the treatment for a few more months and later on try a three-month period without the treatment and see if there is any deterioration. You will then have a good idea of how helpful it is and can restart it if it is beneficial.

It is a good idea to let your GP or consultant know about any supplements, homeopathic or herbal remedies that you are considering as some substances can alter the reactions of other medications that you may be taking and some combinations do not work well together. For instance, homeopathic medicines are not effective when taken with strong-flavoured foods like coffee or peppermint.

There is now more information available on this subject than there has ever been so now is an excellent time to be trying out some complementary approaches. If you would like to learn more please visit www.icnm.org.uk, the Institute for Complementary and Natural Medicine website.

Please see other sections of this book for information on acupuncture, massage and the TENS machines, the Alexander Technique, relaxation, yoga and tai chi. I have also included some useful websites and contact numbers in the Resources section.

Key points

- It is worthwhile to keep informed about the possible benefits of foods and food supplements.
- Nutrition is important and a change of diet may help relieve RA symptoms.
- Other dietary considerations include weight reduction.
- A number of complementary therapies can help to reduce pain.

5

How to Protect Your Joints and Reduce Pain

It's not what you do it's the way that you do it!

Joint protection is an alternative method of carrying out everyday tasks, which will reduce the strain on your joints and therefore reduce pain. Using these techniques will also help to minimise joint deformities. Joint protection is often taught as a group session at an Occupational Therapy department. It involves both formal teaching and practical applications. People often enjoy being in a group as they can then encourage each other and swap ideas. Indeed, it is often the case that this is the first opportunity that people with rheumatoid arthritis have had to talk to others with it.

In order to achieve the optimum results from these sessions it is necessary to incorporate the new ideas on a daily basis. This will take quite a lot of thought initially but later on, if practised regularly, it will become automatic. *If joint protection is incorporated into the daily routine then significant benefits should result.* A study in *The Lancet*[1] in 1991 demonstrated significant improvements in physical abilities for people with rheumatoid arthritis who attended the OT department for a programme of joint protection and other OT interventions.

There are three main principles involved in joint protection as follows.

1   Conserving your energy.
2   Avoiding static positions.
3   Discouraging deformities.

1 Conserving your energy

Having rheumatoid arthritis means that you are likely to have less energy than the average person when the rheumatoid arthritis is active. It also means that your joints are much more vulnerable to damage than other people's joints are. You therefore need to be organised and only do things that are absolutely necessary or things that are important to you. This is particularly necessary if you have a flare-up and feel very tired. How much can be left undone depends on the situation you are in.

It is better to try to organise your life so that on an average day it is possible to fit in everything you want to do with time to spare. This means not taking on too much and being realistic in what you decide to achieve. In fact, this should apply to everyone, not just people with rheumatoid arthritis. Try to spread the workload evenly over the week or month so that there is an even balance of more physical activities and more restful ones. For example, it is not a good idea to clean all the windows on the same day, it is better to do one per day or one a week. Equally, it is not a good choice to sit at a computer all day. Even if you are looking after young children it is possible to vary the activities carried out in any one day and, incidentally, this is much better for the children, too. You can do some physical activities but sit down and enjoy a game or read a book in between the demanding tasks.

Planning and prioritising

Think about the type of work you do because it may be possible to alter the planning of the day or build in rests. It might even be a good idea to change the type of work altogether if it is continually putting strain on the same joints or making you very tired. Start by analysing your working day and deciding what can be eliminated, if anything, and find a beneficial pattern of activity and rest for what remains. Ensure that you do some physical tasks because it is important to exercise to keep muscles strong. It is the balance of activity and rest that is essential. *Prioritise and schedule the most important issues first.* Sometimes we put too high expectations and standards on ourselves. Some tasks can be left undone without it really mattering too much; after all, *health is the most important issue.*

It is also important to think about the way you do tasks and the postures that you adopt for them because you could be placing more strain on your joints or taking more effort than you need to.

- Is there an easier way to carry out this activity?
- Could it be done less often?
- Alternatively could someone else be doing it?

I practise energy conservation and the way I do this is by spreading my work hours over five days and working about five hours daily. I can do this because, luckily, I do not have to work full time. After work and at weekends I tend to do a mixture of physical activities like housework, cooking, walking the dog, swimming, shopping, light gardening and some restful ones like reading, singing, listening to music, telephoning, watching TV, socialising and using the computer. I never do more than two hours of anything and I take coffee breaks frequently! Occasionally I go out for a day and do more walking than usual and often I end up paying the price later in the day or the next day. It is still worth it on the odd occasion if you really want to do something special.

2 Avoiding static positions

A static position is one that involves using the same set of muscles continually rather than alternating the groups of muscles used. For instance, if you sit and hold up a newspaper this places the shoulder muscles in a static position. However, swinging your arms while you are walking is an action that involves continually changing the muscle groups. *It places more strain on a joint to continually use it in the same way and it also uses more energy to maintain a static position.*

Anyone with rheumatoid arthritis needs to continually change positions to avoid repeated strain on particular joints. This means alternating between standing, sitting, walking and lying down. It also means that if you are working using your finger joints then your next action should preferably involve the use of different joints or the same joints used in a different way.

For instance, if you are mixing a cake then this involves a beating motion with the hands and most of the strain is on the elbows, shoulders and wrists, so the next task should use the hands in a different way. You could change to typing because this is using the fingers, wrists and shoulders in a different way, but it would be even better to walk the dog or sit down and read because this would be a complete change of activity involving different joints. Gentle movements of the joints seem to be best because they stop the joints stiffening, but do not strain them. I find that small amounts of light washing up are actually very beneficial. The warm water and gentle movements make the joints feel more comfortable.

Carrying out activities around the house is more beneficial than a long walk, providing they are not too strenuous. This is because the movement loosens the stiffness but does not cause pain. If you need to sit down for a long time then get up and stretch your legs every 20 minutes or so. It is always a good idea to change positions every 20–30 minutes if you are able to.

3 Discouraging deformities

In rheumatoid arthritis the first joints to be affected are usually the fingers, wrists and toes. The overproduction of fluid results in the ligaments becoming loose and then these joints are able to move in an abnormal way. Inflammation sometimes also causes the tendons to weaken. Joint damage means that some movements are restricted.

This restriction, combined with the loose ligaments, weak tendons and the swelling of the joints means that affected joints are then used in abnormal ways to compensate. For instance, if the wrist movement is reduced then finger joints are more likely to take up abnormal positions to counteract this, such as the finger joints drifting and the fingers becoming angled towards the little finger. This is called **ulnar drift** (see Figure 2). Care is needed so that the fingers are not encouraged to take up these positions. Putting pressure on joints also makes deformity more likely.

Joint protection procedures will not stop these things happening but they will slow down the process. Using the joints in as normal a way as possible also means that, if joints do fuse because of cartilage damage, they will fuse in a normal working position and therefore it will still be possible to carry out many actions.

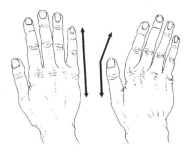

Fig. 2. Normal hand and ulnar drift.

Avoid actions that encourage deformity

Opening jars, screwing lids, turning taps and holding plates can encourage deformities in the hands. You should hold a dinner plate either with two hands or by using the palm of the hand (see Figure 3). It is also better to use the palm of the hand when opening jars or bottles.

If you have to perform a turning or twisting movement using the fingers, always ensure that the fingers are being encouraged to move towards the thumb and not towards the little finger. This means that learning to use both hands is very useful. For example:

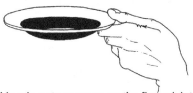

This grip puts pressure on the finger joints
and encourages deformity

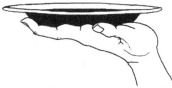

Support the plate on the palm of the hand
if it is not too hot, otherwise use two hands

Fig. 3. Holding a plate.

▓ You should turn on a tap with your right hand and turn it off with your left one.

▓ You could use a special jar opener to open the jar more easily (see Chapter 6).

▓ Use a wall tin opener for tins if they do not have a ring pull opener.

▓ Never pull open ring pull cans with one finger, use a knife to lever them open or use a special ring pull opener.

▓ Finger joints can also be placed into positions of deformity by pushing up on the knuckles or leaning the chin onto the hands. Both these positions should be avoided.

▓ Reading a book by holding it up in one hand can put strain on the finger joints. It is better to rest the book on the table or use a book-rest or draw up the knees and rest it on them.

Avoid tight grips

It places more pressure on the joints to pick up small items than larger ones.

▓ Handles on utensils should be larger to reduce the strain.

▓ It is therefore better to use mugs with thick handles rather than elegant china teacups with dainty handles (see Figure 4).

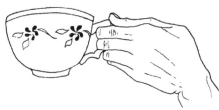

Holding this dainty cup puts pressure on the finger joints

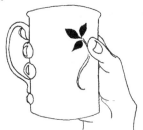

Use a mug with a large handle. Place the fingersaround the mug if it is not too hot

Fig. 4. Holding a drink.

- Spreading your fingers around the mug is a much better position for the finger joints but always wait until the drink has cooled or use an insulated mug.

- Use kitchen tools and cutlery with chunkier handles rather than slim ones.

- If you are using a knife ensure that it is sharp, as this reduces the power needed to cut. There are special knives that can also be used, and these will be discussed in the equipment and adaptations section in Chapter 6.

- Use a thick pen or a pen grip, particularly if you intend to write for long periods of time.

Use a larger joint or several joints rather than small joints

- If you are carrying objects like saucepans and plates then use two hands. Using one hand will place that hand in a position of deformity.

- You can buy two-handled dishes, casseroles and saucepans.

- It is useful to use a tray to carry items but make sure that it has suitable handles at each side.

- It is never a good idea to carry heavy loads and certainly not on one or two fingers. Alternatively they can be carried close to the body in a bag.

- Shopping bags should be carried over the arm or over the shoulder and they should not be too heavy (see Figure 5).

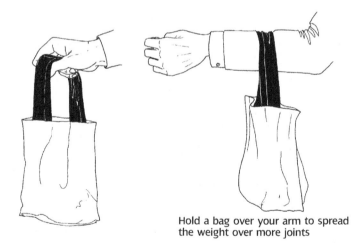

Hold a bag over your arm to spread the weight over more joints

Fig. 5. Holding a shopping bag.

- It is always better to spread loads over more joints or use larger joints.
- Use a car or home delivery wherever possible, or otherwise a trolley, rather than carry weights long distances.

Choose suitable equipment

- Using lightweight equipment will reduce the strain on joints. There are lighter options for most equipment, whether it is for kitchen use, for DIY or for housework. If you are buying new equipment or being given a present, choose with the weight in mind rather than just going for looks.
- Choose fittings that can easily be operated, like levers rather than knobs. For example, choose lever taps in place of crystal or traditional four-prong taps.

A personal scenario

Occupational Therapists will give this information to their clients if they are referred for therapy. I was not referred until I already had many deformities and therefore I did not know about joint protection until I had had rheumatoid arthritis for ten years. I therefore did all the wrong things for a very long time.

As I mentioned, at the time the arthritis started I was working in a park. I was digging, driving a tractor, lifting heavy wheelbarrows and a very heavy teapot. I did not want to appear pathetic and soldiered on even though I was in a lot of pain and my joints were very stiff. It is likely that I would have suffered a lot less pain if I had practised joint protection.

Dr Alison Hammond[2] is an Occupational Therapist who has evaluated joint protection. In 2001 the results of her evaluation of 65 rheumatoid arthritis patients were published. She found significant improvements in pain, disease status and functional ability amongst patients on the joint protection programme.

Liz MacLeod[3] is a physiotherapist who has published guidelines on the pain concern website. She talks about learning to negotiate. She says that some pain sufferers have changed their lifestyle and reduced their flare-ups, whilst others have made little or no changes and endure pain and distress.

I have learnt to negotiate in order that I can be pain free, although this does not mean that I have been prepared to give up everything that I enjoy. There have been many times when I have chosen to ignore joint protection because I had to achieve a personal goal, however I only ignore it for an extremely good reason. At 39 I had never achieved my ambition of going skiing and for a week I put my principles on hold and punished my joints and also risked a few broken bones. I did some exercise before I went and luckily my bones survived intact. It was well worth the risk to achieve an ambition. I really enjoyed the opportunity to ski.

Generally though, since being aware of joint protection, I am a lot more careful. I mostly follow the guidelines and have also found my own ways to make my life easier and to protect my joints. In the kitchen my cooker is near to the sink and I can slide saucepans along. I can then tip them from the edge of the sink into a colander without the need to lift them. I took a lot of care when I bought the cooker, ensuring that I could use the controls. The knobs are an optimum size and easy to turn and the oven is self cleaning inside. These priorities came before being fashionable or having the colour or model that I preferred. Within the price range it usually means that I effectively have very little choice!

All the taps in the house are now very easy to use and if any equipment is due to be replaced I always choose very light items. Most of my pots and pans have two handles or are very light and I am still able to cook the meals. I can also take the vacuum cleaner upstairs, as well as doing the ironing and most light domestic activities.

On the whole, once you have learnt the principles of joint protection you will find ways of incorporating them into your own lifestyle. I have my own way of peeling potatoes. I put them onto the surface, holding them still with one hand and then I use a sharp knife to peel downwards. I do not hold the potatoes in my hand because it is uncomfortable and encourages deformity. I have drawers that can slide open easily and I use appropriate heights to prepare food. I also have a small jug kettle, or otherwise use both hands when I lift a larger kettle. I use a plastic jug to fill the kettle.

Sometimes specialised equipment is necessary to assist with reducing deformities and the reduction of strain on the joints. I have a few items that I regularly use. In the next chapter I will outline the most commonly used equipment that can be beneficial for people with rheumatoid arthritis.

Key points

▶ Learning how to protect your joints will minimise deformities, and reduce strain and pain.

▶ Look at how you can conserve your energy.

▶ Make sure you continually change position, to avoid joint strain.

▶ You can discourage joint deformity by learning practical techniques which avoid stressful actions.

6

Equipment and Adaptations

If there is an easy way to solve a problem why take the hard way?

Equipment is given to people to enable them to do tasks or occupations that they may not otherwise be able to manage independently. This could be because of:

- pain;
- weak muscles; or
- shortness of breath.

Sometimes equipment will be offered to keep someone safe. In the case of people with rheumatoid arthritis the specialised equipment is most often given out in order to protect joints from unnecessary strain. The reduced strain on the joints will help to reduce pain.

A study by Nordenskiold[1] in 1994 reported that pain decreased significantly when the subjects were using assistive devices (disability equipment). The report stated:

assistive devices increase the capacity and the ability to work at home and outside the home.

On the whole many people with rheumatoid arthritis are likely to be apprehensive about using special equipment because they feel labelled as 'disabled' if they use it. Generally speaking, changing the environment, the technique being used or buying useful items that are universally available will be more acceptable. In fact, many items that are useful for people with disabilities would be very useful for other people to use too. The following pages outline some of the most useful items that may be of help to you in your everyday life as well as some suggestions to make life easier for you. Ask your local Social Services or Citizens' Advice Bureau for details of a local disability resource centre or shops that sell disability equipment. Social Services may be able to give you equipment if it is needed for essential activities of daily living.

Equipment for the kitchen

Kitchen equipment is the most usual equipment that you are likely to be offered. This is because almost everyone is involved in drink and meal preparation every day of their lives, so it makes sense to reduce the strain on joints and minimise the likelihood of deformities.

Drink preparation

Use a light kettle or a kettle tipper (see Figure 6) and a light plastic jug to fill the kettle. Use a mug with a substantial handle. Kettle tippers are not always the answer if there are a lot of people sharing the kitchen and they also tend to make people feel disabled. It may be better to have a small or light kettle. Alternatively use two hands to lift the kettle.

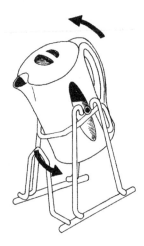

Fig. 6. A kettle tipper.

Meal preparation

■ Ensure knives are sharp. You can use knives with L-shaped handles if you have limited strength (see Figure 7).

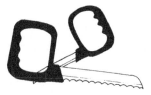

Fig. 7. Knives with L-shaped handles.

■ Choose utensils with wide grip handles, and pans and dishes that are light or double handled. This type of equipment is now more universally available than it used to be when I first needed it. You could use a frying basket to lift vegetables out of the water and then you can empty the saucepan separately when it is lighter. Alternatively you can steam vegetables or put them into the microwave on a light dish.

■ Save the trouble of peeling potatoes by cooking jacket potatoes or boiling potatoes with their skins on. If they need to be peeled use a potato peeler with an enlarged handle or use my method as discussed previously (page 51).

■ Use a wall tin opener or an electric can opener for your tins.

■ There are many bottle and jar openers available but try them out before you purchase any. I have a v-shaped opener that is fitted under a wall cupboard and this has been successful over the years for opening jars and bottles (see Figures 8a and 8b). Ring pull tins may be opened by using a knife as a lever to release the pressure and then by using the knife to assist in levering the lid off. Alternatively turn the tin upside down and use the tin opener or purchase a ring pull opener.

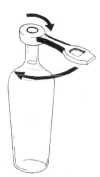

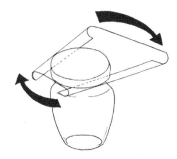

Fig. 8a. A bottle opener which acts as a lever.

Fig. 8b. A v-shaped opener: use both hands to turn the jar and release the lid.

I have also found that a food processor is an essential requirement if you intend to do a lot of chopping and grating. If at all possible, plan the kitchen so that pans can be slid along, to save lifting, and ensure that worktops are the appropriate height for what you are doing. Take care when you are choosing equipment: always try it out as much as possible.

Lastly always have a good pair of scissors handy for all that awkward packaging that is so irritating!

Equipment and tips for personal care

Washing/showering/bathing

Equipment will probably not be needed unless you have problems with your hips and knees or are having a flare-up of your symptoms. In this case you may need some bath equipment. There are many different types of bath-boards and bath-seats available so do your homework thoroughly before purchasing. There are also various types of battery-powered lifts that will allow you to press a button and rise up and down from the bottom of the bath.

A bath is very beneficial when you have rheumatoid arthritis as the warm water relaxes muscles and eases pain. Alternatively use a shower. The effect is not so relaxing but it does keep you clean! A power shower is almost as good as having a bath. It may be difficult to reach around your back so a long-handled sponge or a loofah with handles can be useful.

I have found shampoo blocks are very useful as bottles are sometimes difficult to hold and to open. I tend to use sponges and shower gel to wash with. Sponges are easier to squeeze out and cover all the body much more easily than flannels. Buy shower gel in containers that are easily squeezable or leave bottles upside down, ready for use.

Cleaning teeth

To clean teeth choose a brush with a thick handle or an electric toothbrush. Take care when choosing toothpaste because some tubes and pump action toothpastes are much easier to squeeze than others. You can squeeze out the toothpaste by squeezing the tube with your arm placed on top, if it is painful or difficult to use your fingers.

Shaving

Try out any electric shaver that you intend to buy to ensure that you can manipulate it, or otherwise you could use light plastic disposable razors if this is easier for you.

Make-up

I normally use a make-up sponge as this puts less strain on joints and is also better for the skin. Choose products that have a wide handle and tubes that have larger lids and are easy to squeeze. Alternatively use jars with wide necks.

Clothing

The hands are usually the first joints to be affected by rheumatoid arthritis, and getting dressed may be difficult due to stiffness, pain and weakness. Any damage to joints, especially if there are any deformities, will reduce function because of the loss of the range of movement at the joints. In either case it makes sense to have clothes that are stretchy or loose fitting, and easy to get in and out of. Buttons and zips should be an adequate size to be managed with the least strain on joints. There are gadgets for pulling zips up and down if these are needed; alternatively attach a length of ribbon or cord. Velcro fastenings can be useful although Velcro does wear out more quickly if it has to be opened a lot, for instance Velcro at the opening of trousers. A dressing stick may be useful if it is difficult to get jumpers, tops or coats on and off (see Figure 9).

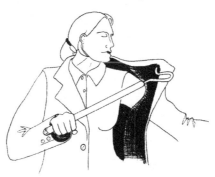

Fig. 9. Using a dressing stick.

It can also be used to pull up socks or reach items that are too high. If you have difficulty bending or need to take precautions following a hip replacement it may be worth trying a sock or stocking aid. This allows you to reach the feet and push the toes into a sock, stocking or tights without the need to bend. These gadgets take time to master but can be helpful once you become skilled at using them.

Shoes

Footwear is very important. Always wear shoes that support the arch and the inside of the foot. If you are going for a long walk then boots or shoes that give good support to the ankle are also a good idea. The sole of the shoe should be capable of cushioning the foot on hard or uneven ground. It will then act as a shock absorber which will help to prevent damage to the joints and will reduce pain in the feet. The heel should always be supported too, otherwise the shoe has to be held in place by the muscles and joints and ligaments of the foot. Socks should be loose fitting so that they do not constrict the circulation, particularly if there is swelling.

If it is uncomfortable or painful to walk then a referral to podiatry (the foot health service) may well be useful. At a foot health department you may have a bio-mechanical assessment. The chiropodist will assess the way that you walk to see how you are using your joints and muscles. Your feet will be examined and then you may be prescribed orthoses (inserts) for your shoes. These will improve the positioning of your feet when you are walking and help to prevent further deformities. They will also make it more comfortable to walk. The chiropodist will also give advice about footwear and foot-care.

I have never been able to wear shoes with heels higher than an inch or two and now I rarely wear tights or stockings. It is just too difficult to put them on and not worth the trouble except for very special occasions. It is a good job that I am happy in trousers with buttoned blouses and tops, which I wear with zipped-up jackets and cardigans. I have to be careful when I am trying them on. I could easily become stuck and unable to get clothes off whilst I am in the fitting room! I always start the selection process by thinking: is the neck big enough? Are the sleeves wide enough? Can I manage the fittings? Is this too tight-fitting for me? After that I can then think about the style and whether it suits me.

I can never understand why so few fitting rooms have chairs or call buttons. Once when I asked for a chair I was told that there was not one in the whole shop. The assistants obviously had to stand all day long.

Selecting furniture

Beds/chairs

As new furniture is purchased ensure that the height of the seat or bed is appropriate for you so that you can get on and off without struggling and putting a strain on the knee and hip joints.

- Chair and bed raisers can be used to raise the existing furniture if this is necessary.
- The toilet should also be an adequate height and many are made too low. If it is a struggle to get off then a raised toilet seat can be fitted. Alternatively, toilets can be raised on plinths, however this is a lot more expensive.

Taps and fittings

- Lever taps are best and these can be purchased in most general DIY stores.
- Ensure washers are changed regularly and taps are not turned off too tightly.
- Lever handles are always more suitable than knobs for all your doors.
- Ensure that any drawers run in and out easily.
- Plugs on vacuum cleaners and irons that are used frequently should be changed for plugs with handles (see Figure 10). These will protect joints and make it easier to pull the plugs out.

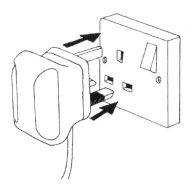

Fig. 10. A plug pull: this plug has an integral handle.

▓ If keys or doorknobs are difficult for you to manage then key turners or knob turners can be bought to give more leverage (see Figures 11 and 12).

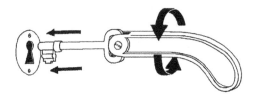

Fig. 11. A key turner: the extended handle is easier to turn.

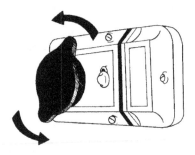

Fig. 12. A knob turner: the larger knob is easier to turn.

▓ Choose phones that are easy to hold, with buttons that can easily be depressed.

▓ Use pens with wide handles or use a pen grip. Writing with a standard pen can put a lot of strain on finger joints if you do a lot of writing.

Adaptations

If you think that you may need adaptations to your home you could request an assessment by an Occupational Therapist. You will need to contact Social Services if you are seeking funding or advice from an OT. A grant may then be available for necessary and appropriate adaptations, although it is likely to be means tested and this means that many young working people are usually ineligible. In council housing these adaptations are presently provided without a means test (in my own area) if they are necessary and appropriate. Some authorities also have schemes for lending money if the means test has eliminated you from obtaining a grant. Low-cost adaptations like grab rails or steps may be provided without a means test. Different councils and county councils have different rules, so you will have to investigate.

Kitchen adaptations are most commonly provided for clients with rheumatoid arthritis. These could be alterations to worktops or cupboards, or changing unsuitable handles, taps or plug points. In the bathroom the most frequent adaptations would be the provision of a shower or providing a seat for a shower, lever taps or hand rails. Another common adaptation is the provision of a stair-lift if someone finds that it is very painful and difficult to go up and down the stairs. Rails of all kinds, such as banister rails, are regularly provided by Social Services and can be very useful for maintaining independence or keeping people safe.

Some people with disabilities are not very happy to have any adaptations that make them feel disabled, and it is also important to maintain muscle strength and keep the joints moving. *It really comes down to weighing up the potential benefits of activity against possible joint damage as well the need to be safe.* For example, if someone can manage stairs safely and without too much pain it is probably better to manage without an extra banister rail or stair-lift unless there is a lot of joint damage to the hips and knees or the person is at risk of falling down the stairs. If an activity is carried out repeatedly, or is very painful, then aids and adaptations are very useful. Otherwise it is important to keep the joints moving and take exercise. The next section examines the value of exercise and the importance of good posture.

Key points

- ▶ Joint strain – and pain – can be reduced by using specialised equipment.
- ▶ You may be reluctant to use special items, but changes to the environment, techniques or equipment can make a difference.
- ▶ Look at changes you might make in the kitchen, personal care and furniture.
- ▶ Consider adaptations to your home – an Occupational Therapist can advise.

7

The Importance of Exercise and Good Posture

There is a delicate balance between doing too much and doing too little.

These days we are continually reminded about the need to exercise in order to keep fit and healthy. This is particularly necessary for people who have a sedentary lifestyle. Anyone who is over the age of 40 needs to take exercise regularly in order to maintain their muscle strength and reduce the risk of osteoporosis. This is even more essential for those of us who have rheumatoid arthritis because we need strong muscles to support our joints, particularly if they are damaged due to cartilage erosion. There are three types of exercise that everyone needs.

Strengthening exercises

These exercises are needed to maintain some muscle strength and if possible to increase it. People with RA need to take care with this type of exercise and the best way to gain muscle strength is to do an exercise class like pilates or tai chi or yoga. If you attend classes you will need to find a practitioner who is sympathetic towards people who have a chronic condition so that there is some flexibility, making it possible to drop in and out of exercises according to joint pain and/ or damage. Once you have the basics it's possible to carry out the exercises at home. However, having a regular class to attend helps to ensure that the exercise continues. You could also request some physiotherapy and continue the exercises yourself at home but again keeping up exercises regularly is difficult to maintain.

Tai chi was evaluated in 2007 in a study that considered 45 studies for the research. Two randomised clinical trials (RCTs) and three non-randomised controlled clinical trials (CCTs) met all the inclusion criteria. 'Two random clinical trials (RCTs) reported some positive findings for tai chi on disability index, quality of life, depression and mood for RA patients.'[1]

A new study outlined on the NRAS website found that people who took part in a strength training programme benefited from a 53% reduction in pain and a 46% improvement in strength.

2 Aerobic or endurance exercise

This type of exercise is needed to maintain and improve cardiovascular fitness and to help control weight. Try any activity that speeds up your heart rate. It does not matter what activity you choose but ensure that you wear shock-absorbent trainers to protect your feet. You need to start with a couple of minutes at a time and gradually increase the time you spend. You might like to try dancing, a racquet sport, cycling or even trampolining. Choose something that you can manage but also enjoy. If you do not enjoy it you are unlikely to continue.

There is also a new option that can help you to exercise if you are limited by joint damage or mobility problems and this is the Wii. You could try either the Wii Sports or the Wii Fit/Wii fit plus. This equipment is a great way to get some aerobic exercise and have fun too. You can do it on your own or with others. You can do yoga, jogging, aerobics, step dancing, virtual hula-hooping, boxing, skateboarding, skiing, slalom, kung fu, to name just a few. It really gets your heart rate going and exercising with others is fun.

3 Range-of-motion exercise

All joints need to be put through their natural range of movement daily, preferably a few times a day, and ideally this should be incorporated into your daily routine. Any exercise that is incorporated into daily life is much more likely to happen. We all know how people sign up at fitness centres in January and stop two months later. The same will apply with sets of exercises; people always mean to do them and start off remembering for a couple of weeks, then they forget.

Planning your exercise

Work out a way of planning the exercise so that it can easily be fitted into your day. This can be done by having a set of exercises to do when you are sitting down at a table, others for when you are in a car in traffic and another set for when you are relaxing in an easy chair. Alternatively you could get into a pattern of:

- doing yoga each day;
- swimming regularly; or
- doing aqua-aerobic exercises in the water.

These three activities are useful because you can go at your own pace in a way that suits your needs without a need to compete. All three allow you to put all your joints through their complete range of movements.

- You could try a gym but take care that your programme is appropriate for you. Always show it to a Physiotherapist or an Occupational Therapist or your GP and discuss the type of exercise that will be beneficial for you.
- Walking is also good exercise. It can be just short distances to the post-box or to a friend's house, or it could be a little dog-walking or shopping where there are only a few light items to carry.
- Cycling can also be good exercise, but again not for too long or it can put a strain on the shoulders, wrists and fingers as well as your knees and hips.
- If you are using the last two activities you will also need exercises for the hands and wrists.

Finding a balance

You need to be able to maintain or improve muscle strength without damaging your joints. You also need to be able to stretch the tendons and ligaments as well as putting each joint through its natural range of movement as far as is possible without pain. It is always a question of finding a balance, varying the joints that you are using and not holding any position for too long.

Do not do anything strenuous and listen to your own body. Always start with short gentle exercise and build up slowly. If you are not able to do some of the exercises just do what you are able to manage.

If you have other medical conditions apart from rheumatoid arthritis talk to your GP first and find out how much exercise is beneficial. If you have a medical condition that affects your heart or lungs this will obviously make exercise more difficult.

Exercise at the table

The following set of exercises was given to me when I first attended Occupational Therapy. The local OT unit still uses most of these exercises.

These exercises will be beneficial for the hands and wrists. They should be performed slowly, stretching as much as possible. Relax between repetitions and gradually increase the repetitions. Reduce the repetitions if your hands hurt.

1   Rest the forearm on the table. Curl your fingers up gently into a fist then gradually uncurl.

2   Place your hands palms down onto the table with the fingers stretched out. Walk your fingers towards the thumb.

3   Hold your hands out in front of you and touch each fingertip onto the thumb. Now touch the base of each finger with the thumb.

4   Hold your hands out in front of you. Have the fingers make a loose fist then circle the hand at the wrist clockwise and anticlockwise and then up and down.

5   Press hands and forearms flat on the table, palms down. Lift up the thumb ... hold ... and then ... down. Repeat with all the fingers and the other thumb.

6   Start as for 5 then roll hands over trying to touch the table with the tips of the thumbs. Roll back to starting position.

7   Put one hand and forearm flat on the table, place the other hand on top. The hand on top will help to straighten out the fingers of the hand underneath. Repeat with the other hand.

8   Put an envelope or a piece of thin card between your thumb and index finger. Try to pull it away with the other hand whilst resisting with your thumb and index finger. Repeat this with the other fingers and the other hand.

Useful yoga exercises

While I have been writing this book I have looked for research to support my ideas. Until the last few years there has been little or no research on complementary approaches to illness, so there are few studies on these topics in relation to rheumatoid arthritis. As far as yoga goes I have found a study by Dr Ian Haslock[2] in which he concluded that rheumatoid arthritis patients could gain definite benefits from yoga. The benefits included reduced pain, increased mobility, increased energy, and reduced tension and stress.

Yoga is an appropriate way to maintain a good range of movements in all your joints. It is a form of exercise that is not competitive and all the moves are done gently and gradually. Yoga helps to strengthen muscles and increase flexibility. Any good yoga book or yoga teacher will advise beginners to exercise for short periods at a time and to stop if there is pain. You will be able to find a selection of moves that will exercise different parts of the body. Remember that if you have rheumatoid arthritis it is not advisable to hold static positions for too long; five to ten seconds will be enough. Never do the exercises if your joints are inflamed. During a flare-up rest is best, or otherwise only very gentle exercise.

Here is a selection of moves that I have found useful over the years. These can be found in any basic yoga book but it is a good idea to begin by attending a yoga class as an introduction to this form of exercise. It is easier to learn initially from a teacher and then use a book to help you carry on with the exercises at your own pace. It is advisable to make the teacher aware of any problems that you may have, e.g. pain or reduced range of movements. In fact most teachers will probably ask about medical conditions as a matter of course. You will also need to bear in mind joint protection techniques. The teacher may be able to help you to formulate a personal exercise plan. There are different forms of yoga, some of which place more emphasis on meditation while others focus more on exercising the body. All forms will teach yoga positions and all of the tutors will be able to recommend suitable books.

Ankle bends

This exercise relieves swollen ankles and feet, improves circulation and removes fatigue in the legs.

Stand with your feet apart. Roll onto the sides of your feet. Roll your feet outwards and then inwards.

The blade

This relieves tension in the shoulders and upper back and can relieve arthritic pain. It also stretches the shoulder joints.

Bend your elbows and bring your fingertips together so that they touch in front of the chest. Now draw your shoulder blades together. Hold for five seconds and release slowly.

The flower

This improves flexibility and reduces stiffness in the fingers.

Make your hands into a fist and open your fingers, gently resisting while you do it, like a flower opening in the morning. Release.

Now stretch your fingers open and gradually close into a fist, again resisting while you do it.

Gently move your fingers or shake your wrist.

Hands to wall

This strengthens the arms and wrists and releases tension in the shoulders.

Stand straight, facing a wall about an arm's length away. Place your palms against the wall with the fingers almost touching. Slowly bend your elbows. Press your palms against the wall and lean forward, resisting all the while until your forehead is against the wall. Hold for five seconds and return just as slowly.

Posture clasp

This improves the posture and eases tension in the shoulders. It also maintains the flexibility of the shoulder joints and strengthens the arms.

Try to bring your left arm up your back as far as it will go with the palm facing out. Lift your right hand straight up above your head, bend the elbow and bring this hand towards the centre of your back.

Try to grasp your left hand by inching your hands gradually together. Hold for a few seconds then gently release. Reverse the hands.

Sitting warrior

This relieves pain in the heels and knees. It is beneficial to prevent fallen arches and flat feet common in rheumatoid arthritis patients.

Kneel in an upright position with your knees together and your feet about half a metre apart. Slowly lower your body to sit between your feet. Keep your back straight and your toes pointed. Relax down. If this hurts too much then sit with your ankles crossed. Gradually over a period of time try to do the exercise with your feet further apart. Alternatively you could place a cushion on your feet and sit on that.

The tree

This will improve circulation and balance. It also encourages good posture and tones the leg muscles.

Stand with your feet together and your arms by your side. Bend your right leg so that the sole of the foot rests against your left thigh. Slide your foot onto your thigh. Your heel should be as high as possible up your thigh. Bring your arms up over your head so that the palms come together. Hold for about ten seconds or as long as balance permits. Lower your legs and hands slowly.

I have chosen a selection of yoga exercises that are beneficial for the hands and feet, shoulders and knees. These are the most commonly affected joints in rheumatoid arthritis. These exercises will help to maintain a good range of movement in these joints. Try to exercise daily.

The following exercises have been adapted from yoga exercises and simplified. They are easier to do if you have a lot of joint damage.

Exercises for the car

These can be done when the car is stopped in a queue or perhaps when you are parked and waiting for someone.

Neck exercises

1   Gently and gradually stretch the neck back and then forward, down onto the chest and back to the normal position.

2   Now gently and slowly turn to the left and then to the right and back to centre.

Exercises for the shoulders
1   Lift the shoulders and roll them up and outwards.
2   Hold the steering wheel with an arm holding each side of the wheel. Have the arms at full stretch and push for a few seconds.

Exercises for the chair

Ankle exercises
Stretch the feet out in front of you and circle the feet outwards and then inwards. Now stretch the toes as far forward as you can to the floor. Now bring the toes up as far as you can.

Hand exercises
Place the forearms on the arms of the chair, hands free over the edge with palms down and the fingers relaxed. Lift hands up ... hold ... put hands down.

Standing exercises
You can do these when, for instance, waiting for a kettle to boil.

Shoulder exercises
1   Start with the hands at the side and then bring each hand as far as you can up your back, palm outwards.
2   Now start with your arms above your head, hands together. Bring your arms outwards and gradually down to your sides. Do one hand at a time if this is easier. You can reverse this if possible and start with the arms at the sides and bring them slowly out and up until they touch together over the head.

Elbow exercises
1   Put your hands behind your head and circle your elbows.
2   Put your hands into loose fists. Touch them together in front of you at chest height. Now stretch both arms out from the elbows as far as you can and in again.

3   Touch your fingertips onto your shoulders then stretch them out to the front and then open the arms out to the sides.

Exercises at the kitchen sink

1   Gently open and close your fingers when washing up and wriggle them around in the water.
2   Bring the palms up and down a few times keeping the wrists still.

Exercises on the bed

1   Lie flat on your back with arms at your side. Now reach your arms up and back so that they lie flat with your hands above your head. Bring them slowly down.
2   Lie on your front with your arms by your sides. Now lift your head and shoulders gently up and back, hold and gradually lie down again.
3   In the same position turn your head to one side, back to the centre and then to the other side to exercise your neck.

Exercises for the bath

Exercise for the arms and shoulders
Sit with your forearms on the edges of the bath. Gently lift yourself up from the water and down again. You could also do the neck exercises as above.

Exercise for the fingers and wrist
Sit with your hands on your thighs. Have the palms flat down and your fingers spread out. Press gently down on your thighs and then relax.

You can also do the shoulder exercise as above (see standing exercises) or the ankle exercises (see exercises for the chair).

Hydrotherapy and swimming

Exercise in the water is very beneficial for people with rheumatoid arthritis because you can put the joints through a full range of movements while the water supports your joints. This means that the exercise is safe for you. Swimming will also maintain muscle strength and if you are able to swim at speed this will also benefit the heart and lungs.

Hydrotherapy is therapy in the water – i.e. exercise in the water – and this is also excellent for increasing the range of movements at the joints and reducing pain. Physiotherapy departments sometimes have a hydrotherapy pool and you may be able to have sessions there if your GP refers you. Our local hydrotherapy pool has a weekly session for arthritis patients. You can start with hydrotherapy if your joints are very painful because the water is warmer than in most swimming pools and this is why it is good for pain relief. If you are able to join a health club with a pool the water will normally be warmer than council pools and it will also be less crowded which means that it is much easier to exercise.

Arthritis Care Research published the results of a controlled trial of hydrotherapy for rheumatoid arthritis in 1996.[3] In this clinical trial patients showed improvements in both physical and psychological measures after the four-week sessions and at the three-month follow-up. Women also had improvements in joint tenderness and range of movements at the knee. Here are some exercises that I do in the swimming pool.

Exercises in the water

1   Lie on your back with your hands at your sides then stretch them up and out so that they touch over your head.
2   Walk on your toes or do the ankle exercises. Try to run through the water.
3   Try to do all the different strokes – i.e. breaststroke, crawl, backstroke, sidestroke, doggy paddle and butterfly – if you are able to as they all exercise different joints.
4   Use a float and stretch your arms out in front of you.
5   With your feet apart try doing 'squats' in the water. Hold the position for the count of five.
6   March through the water swinging your arms and lifting your knees.

In fact you can do any of the standing exercises in the water. Alternatively go to an aqua-aerobics class.

The benefits of exercise

I have looked at research to find out what proven benefits exercise has shown for people with rheumatoid arthritis. A working party of the Royal College of Physicians[4] convened in 1989 and they examined the evidence for regular exercise. They made several recommendations for their members. Their conclusions were that there is now good evidence of many physical and psychological benefits to the general population in taking regular exercise. They recommended that doctors should check if patients are taking exercise and then advise patients on the extent and type of activity suitable for each individual. They also stated that exercise should start in childhood and continue into old age wherever possible.

In 1994 P.H. Fentem[5] wrote 'The benefits of exercise in health and disease'. He said that people with disabilities were prone to inactivity and this must not be accepted as normal. He mentioned the deleterious effects of inactivity and stated that the benefits of exercise could mean a return to work for people with rheumatoid arthritis who had previously given up their jobs due to ill health.

An article on the ARC website[6] contains an interview with Kathleen Turner who has rheumatoid arthritis. In the article Kathleen explains that her doctor told her:

> *Get into the pool no matter how much it hurts, no matter how little you can do, but keep moving.*

She goes on to say that this is the best thing for her, better than any drug. She has to keep moving. I agree with Kathleen Turner: it is very important to keep moving. It prevents the joints feeling stiff and maintains the muscle strength. It is still important to balance activities and it is still necessary to rest when there is an acute flare-up but generally *keep moving* is a good motto.

A personal scenario

You need to be able to find a way of exercising which suits you and hopefully that you also enjoy. I have never had a problem with taking exercise as I have always enjoyed sports like badminton, walking, swimming, etc. The main problem that I have had to deal with is the deterioration of my joints over many years. Activity and exercise does not stop the disease, it only helps by maintaining muscle strength and keeping a good range of movement at all the joints for as long as possible. If muscles are not used they will waste and strong muscles help to support the joints. This is particularly important where there is joint damage.

The problems that I have had to face in the past include having to play badminton with no wrist movement (and that is certainly not ideal!), having to change my three-mile walks to shorter bird-watching rambles, swimming at half my previous speed and strength and not being able to play tennis.

I am not a very competitive person but it can be frustrating at times. Some people prefer not to do things at all if they cannot do them extremely well. In this case they may well find that they need to give up certain pastimes and find a new challenge. I always chose to carry on while I could still enjoy the activity. I do not play badminton any more because I cannot run and in the past I had to give up tennis because the racquet was too heavy for me (although racquets are now much lighter than they used to be). My yoga abilities have also diminished. I used to be able to do the lotus but now I am lucky if I can do a few stretches. I do enjoy my swimming though. It allows my joints to feel much more mobile and the jacuzzi afterwards is a reward for the exercise before!

I will never know how much the exercise has helped me but I do feel that it is of great value both in maintaining my physical functioning as well as my mental health, given the severe joint damage that I have suffered over the years.

Good posture

As well as doing exercise it is important to ensure that you have good posture. This is particularly important for anyone with rheumatoid arthritis because the pain or discomfort that occurs tends to make you avoid certain positions and movements. This means that if, for instance, your right foot hurts then you will put more weight on the left one, or if your neck hurts you may hold your head in a tilted position without realising it. In either case the body is not working in its natural way and the spine will be compensating to keep the body in balance. This can cause back problems and/or damage to the joint that is working harder, such as the left foot or the neck in the instances above.

Avoidance of any particular movement for prolonged periods means that the ligaments and tendons in the affected area will shorten because they are not being used fully. This means, for instance, that if you were to remain sitting in a wheelchair for months and you never straightened your legs out, the tendons would gradually shorten and the knees would become contracted and then it would become impossible to stand. This is why it is vital to put all joints through their normal range of movements (or as much as you can manage) regularly and to try as far as possible to ensure correct posture at all times. A Physiotherapist or Occupational Therapist will be able to give advice on this.

Alexander Technique

Alternatively it may be worth paying privately for a practitioner who can advise you on the Alexander Technique, particularly if bad habits have already been practised for a long time.

The Alexander Technique teaches you to be aware of your body and to think about the way that you are carrying out physical actions. The practitioner will guide you and make you aware of incorrect postures and in this way you will improve the body's alignment. This will then prevent bad posture, muscle tension and pain.

Guidelines for good posture

Here are some general guidelines to follow.

Standing

Figure 13a illustrates good posture and the following text summarises how to achieve this.

■ Always ensure that your head is not tilted to the left or to the right, forwards or backwards. Look in the mirror to make sure you are looking straight ahead. If your head is carried correctly then it is more likely that weight will be spread through your body correctly.

■ If your weight is not distributed properly this will place a strain on your joints. Stand so that your weight is placed equally through both feet.

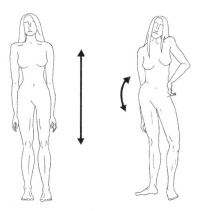

Fig. 13a. Good standing posture.   **Fig. 13b. Bad posture.**

▪ The ankles, knees, hips and shoulders should be in line when standing.

▪ Do not stand for too long.

Figure 13b is an extreme example of bad posture, demonstrating how not to stand. The head is tilted, the weight is on one side, the body is twisted and the shoulder joint is dropped on one side. The weight is distributed unevenly and the joints are under strain.

Walking

▪ Wear supportive shoes that give arch support and support to the inside of the foot.

▪ Push off from the heels and roll onto the toes.

▪ Try to keep a spring in the step if at all possible.

▪ Do not walk with the head down. Ensure the head is in a balanced position as in standing.

Sitting

▪ Sit on a chair of the correct seat height so that your back is supported and your feet are flat on the floor.

▪ An armrest and headrest are useful.

▪ You should sit up straight and not slump down, however you should relax the shoulders. See Figures 14a and 14b, showing good and bad sitting posture.

▪ It is important to choose furniture that is supportive, firm and comfortable.

■ If you have short legs you may find that many chairs have too great a distance from the back to the front of the seat, and it is therefore difficult to support your back and reach the floor without curving your back. Shop around and find one that is suitable, it will be well worth it.

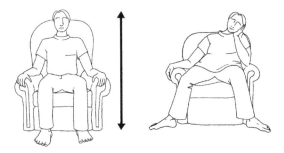

Fig. 14a. Good sitting posture.   Fig. 14b. Poor sitting posture.

Lying down

■ Have a mattress that is firm but also feels soft.

■ Use a pillow that just cushions the curve at the neck. It should not be too high and you should not use two unless you have some sort of breathing problems.

■ Ensure that the bed is of an appropriate height to get in and out of easily. This will prevent strain on the knees and hips when you get out.

Working at a worktop or desk

See Figures 15a and 15b demonstrating correct and incorrect posture when seated at a desk.

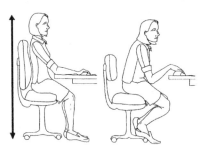

Fig. 15a. Correct working posture.   Fig. 15b. Incorrect working posture.

■ The desk should be of an appropriate height so that you do not have to lean forward. Your arm should be supported when writing.

■ A speakerphone is essential if you have to do a lot of phone work.

■ Worktops should be of an appropriate height. You need the surface lower for hard work, such as mixing a cake, but higher for chopping and lighter work.

Whatever you are doing remember to change positions frequently. You should not sit at a keyboard for more than 20–30 minutes. Stand up and walk across the office, stretch your fingers, etc. This will prevent you from getting stiff and will allow you to move more easily.

If you have unsuitable furniture and equipment at your workplace you could give Access to Work a try. This is a scheme that can be used to fund adaptations to your workplace if you have a disability (details in Chapter 9).

The good posture habit

It does seem that there is a lot to remember, but if you remind yourself to think about your posture for a few weeks then you will easily get into the habit of good posture. It will be time well spent if it reduces joint damage and pain.

Key points

▶ Exercise is very important – you need strong muscles to support joints.

▶ Work out an exercise plan to fit into your day.

▶ Find a balance: start with gentle exercise and build up slowly.

▶ Good posture is also important to keep the body in balance.

8

How to Relax and Manage Your Stress

There are only two ways to handle tense situations; you can change them or you can change the way you look at them. (Wilson)[1]

This chapter looks at the link between pain, tension and stress. I will look at how to reduce pain by relaxation and give a taster of some relaxation exercises.

Although a lot of research has been done to try to find out if stress is a trigger for the onset of chronic diseases, or if stress causes flare-ups for existing conditions, it is still not clear if indeed there is a link. Research appears to indicate different conclusions. The reason that these results are inconclusive may be because it is not only the amount of stress that you have to deal with that is important, but also the way that the stress is dealt with.

We all have some stress in our lives and, in fact, we all need a certain level of stress to function at our optimum level. Stress is often considered to be about having lots to do and having deadlines to complete tasks, but although this can be stressful it is also this stress that gives us the urgency to get started. We all know that if you have too much time you tend to continually procrastinate and leave things for another day. It is always said that if you need something done quickly then ask a busy person! Yet we all vary in the amount of stress that we can manage and therefore we all have to learn how much we can cope with successfully. *To do this we need to learn to notice the symptoms of stress that occur when we have too much to manage.*

Sometimes it is easier for other people to notice the signs of stress than it is for us to realise ourselves that we are under too much stress. We need to become better at noticing the symptoms and taking action.

The signs that indicate that we are not coping are unique to each individual, but there are lots of common features and we are all likely to exhibit some of them. The signs of stress can be divided into different categories:

- physical;
- cognitive; and
- behavioural symptoms.

Symptoms of Stress

1 Physical symptoms
These are the ones that we can feel:

- headaches;
- tense stomach or feeling sick;
- sweating;
- raised heartbeat;
- sleeplessness.

2 Cognitive symptoms
These ones affect our thinking:

- difficulties in concentrating;
- negative thoughts;
- mental blocks;
- finding difficulty in making a decision;
- feeling guilty when you are not doing anything.

3 Behavioural symptoms
These are the ones that change our behaviour:

- impatience;
- short temper;
- aggression;
- eating too much or too little;
- irritability;
- frustration;
- smoking and drinking to excess;
- tearfulness.

A definition of stress

These are the most common symptoms of stress but what exactly is stress? It is a word that is used very frequently and in many different ways. The word was originally used in engineering terms to mean a force that could be applied to a structure until it would collapse. In human terms it has a similar meaning – in other words there is only so much stress that we can stand before we suffer a breakdown. If there is too much pressure in our situation for us to deal with, then we can no longer perform at our optimum level. The point at which this is reached will be different for everyone, although the situations that cause us to be stressed will be similar.

Why stress occurs

Stress normally builds up when there is too much uncertainty in our lives and not necessarily because we have a lot to do. It could be because there are important decisions to be made in connection with work or family issues, and these decisions are difficult and we are putting them off. It could be because there is too much to do and not enough time to do it in and it is difficult to know what to do first. Sometimes we feel burdened by conflicting roles and we feel as though we cannot manage them all.

Another reason for stress could be that we feel inadequate because we cannot do anything as well as we would like and we feel that we are failing others or ourselves. Once there is too much pressure things will inevitably start going wrong and more crises will happen. At this point the correct balance for our own body needs to be restored or we become in danger of a complete breakdown of health (see Figure 16).

It can be seen from this diagram of the human function curve that performance gets better with some stress, but eventually there is too much arousal. At this point we need to restore the balance. It can also be seen that it is possible to have too little arousal because of too little stimulation and then performance is also poor. Whatever the situation we need to maintain a balance. This is important for everyone, but especially for those of us with rheumatoid arthritis because the stress may well be making our condition worse.

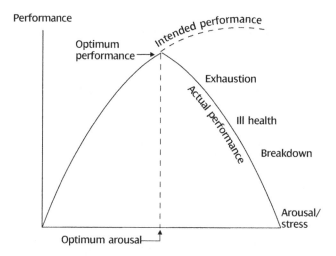

Fig. 16. Human function curve.

Restoring the balance

Often if we are unable to cope it is because we have taken on too much. We have done this either because we have underestimated how long things will take or because we were unable to say no. It is crucial to decide what is important for us to do and what we can let go of. At college I worked through a very useful exercise that can be used to help people to decide which activities and roles they would like to carry on with and which are dispensable. It is called the **juggling act**. You imagine yourself as a juggler and at the start of the exercise you will be holding too many balls to manage. You will need to decide which balls you will hold onto and which you will let go of. You may need a friend or relative to help you with this because the more stressed you are the more difficult it is to make decisions. Having made the decision you must then carry it through. To do this you may need to be assertive.

Being assertive

This is another word that tends to be used a lot these days and it is often confused with being aggressive. Being assertive means being responsible for making your own decision and carrying it out. It means stating your intentions without getting angry or upset. It involves making clear statements about the way you feel or what you intend to do, but always respecting other people's feelings and rights. It means recognising your own needs and wants and doing something about them.

If you are not assertive you will tend to let others make decisions for you or you will give up easily. You will be very bad at saying no and therefore will end up doing things that you really do not want to do. This can then make you feel angry, frustrated or worn out from doing too much.

If you feel that you are not assertive enough then it would definitely be beneficial for you to go on an assertiveness course. These may be offered to you in your work environment but otherwise you can contact the local education authority or college. I was not very assertive in my teens and twenties but I attended a course when I was in my late thirties and I found it extremely useful. It helped me to say no and to act to resolve problems and express my feelings more clearly to others. This is very important if you have rheumatoid arthritis because you will need to be able to let others know about any help that you require. You may need to negotiate changes at work (see Chapter 9) and you will definitely need to make decisions in relation to your medical condition. It is also a good idea to do as much as you can to reduce stress because it may be aggravating your medical condition.

Decision making

Failing to make a decision is another reason that makes us suffer stress. This happens either because we are putting off making a decision that needs to be made or because there is too much uncertainty surrounding the issue for a decision to be made. If it is the latter then you either need to look at all the different scenarios and make a number of alternative plans, or you need to learn to switch this problem off for the time being until it is possible to make the decision. It is no use worrying about things before they happen. The decisions can be made when the time comes.

Alternatively take action to obtain the information you need so that you will be able to make the decision. If a decision needs to be made and you have all the information to do this, and the situation is unlikely to change, then do it straight away. Write down the pros and cons and choose. Get someone to assist if you like. You will feel a whole lot better when the decision is made and carried out.

Decisions are usually made by intuition rather than logic. However, it is often necessary to go through the pros and cons before you realise what you really wanted the decision to be. If you have ever flipped a coin in order to decide something, you will know that the choice from the coin toss either confirms your decision or makes you choose the other option. This is because the coin toss has made you aware of what you had already decided on but would not admit, or it has made you choose what you were not consciously aware of. So it can still be helpful to go through the process in order to get the decision made. Sometimes you just know what to do and in this case you can go ahead, there is no need to wait.

The longer the indecision goes on, the worse you will feel. After you have made the decision remind yourself about all the good reasons that led you to making it and all the benefits that the decision has given you. Once decisions have been made and plans carried out then the symptoms of stress will gradually reduce, although it may take your body a few days or weeks to get back to normal.

The fight or flight response

You can begin to reduce the physical symptoms of stress by relaxation techniques. Physical symptoms of stress arise because the body reacts to stress in the same way that it would react to being chased by a tiger. It prepares for **fight or flight**. This means that if you were in a situation where you had to fight or run away your body would prepare for action. In order to have increased energy, and so that your muscles would be ready to begin running, your body would prepare in the following way. There would be an increase in heart rate and blood pressure, extra production of adrenalin, your metabolic rate would increase and so would the blood flow to the muscles. More sweat would be produced and your muscles would become tense. At the same time the digestive system and the immune system would be subdued so that the body could put all its energy into the fight or flight.

The body reacts in exactly the same way in order to combat stress. If the body continually acts in this state of preparation because of stress, then it never gets a chance to recover. It is always in a state of alert and it is never resting. *The immune system and the digestive system will become less efficient so it is essential to relax.*

Learning to relax

We need to learn to relax so that the body can recharge itself, energy levels are restored and there is a feeling of well-being. Having your body wound up into a state of tension uses a lot of energy. During relaxation there is a reduction of breathing rate, heart rate, blood flow and muscle action and a lowering of the hormones that cause these actions. The body is therefore able to restore itself. During relaxation the brain produces alpha rhythms instead of beta rhythms: alpha rhythms have a therapeutic effect in the restoration of bodily health.

Relaxation is a skill that has to be learnt and it takes time and practice. It is probably better to go on a course or have individual lessons when you begin learning. There now many more complementary health centres and these usually offer relaxation courses. Alternatively, speak to your GP or visit the type of shop that specialises in gems, crystals and rocks, as these often have this type of course available. These shops also sell relaxation tapes or CDs of relaxing music and sound compilations. If you are self disciplined and determined you may be able to learn by using tapes or CDs or by recording your own script.

To practise you will need to find a comfortable place with no disturbance in order to achieve relaxation, but as you get better you will learn to relax yourself anywhere at any time. You will become aware of your body and you will recognise symptoms of anxiety and stress and you will be able to control them.

The postures of stress

Learn to become aware of certain postures which indicate that you are tense or under stress.

Head

Forwards or downwards with the chin tucked in. If this position is held for long it can lead to neck and head pain.

Arms

Shoulders are hunched up. Elbows bent and arms held into the body.

Hands

Fingers are closed into a fist or objects are gripped tightly. There could be continual fiddling with an object such as a pen or ring.

Legs

If seated, legs will be crossed or wound around each other and if the person is sitting on a seat they will sit on the edge of it.

If standing, the person moves around a lot, or changes legs, or crosses and uncrosses the legs continually.

Body

Stooped forward or held rigidly. A continual posture of stress can cause back pain.

Face

Jaw clamped shut, lips tightly closed, the teeth may grind. Brows and eyes screwed up.

Any of these positions can lead to pain.

Getting started

This section is a brief look at breathing, and relaxing the body and mind. It is beneficial to learn in a class or obtain a tape, CD or book for more details.

At the beginning of a relaxation session always take a couple of relaxing breaths first to ease tension. You also need to ensure that you are comfortable, so have a fidget around first before settling down.

The following extract from a progressive passive relaxation exercise is one that I have often used and found helpful. It was given to me by a hypnotherapist. I feel that this type of exercise is better for people with painful joints as it does not involve any tensing up of muscles. You just focus on your breathing and the different parts of the body in turn and let go of tension. I have a selection of different relaxation exercises that I learnt on my OT training course. I have listened to them all and found my own way of relaxing. You will need to find a method that you are happy with yourself. The voice on tapes can be very relaxing for you or it might be very irritating – find one that works to relax you.

Passive progressive relaxation

Make yourself as comfortable as you can by stretching and getting into a good position. Notice if you are clenching or tightening your muscles. Let your arms, legs and whole body go floppy. Gently close your eyes. Use a few long, deep breaths to breathe out all the tension. Hold a deep breath in for a few seconds and breathe out. Repeat this a few times, relaxing your body with each out breath. If you hear sounds around you use them to help you to relax. Let them recede into the distance as you relax into your breathing. Notice the rise and fall of your chest. Breathe easily and freely relaxing more and more as you breathe out.

After this the next stage is to go through all the parts of the body, either starting at the feet and going up, or at the head and working down. You need to become aware of each part of the body and release the tension in each part. You should begin to feel warm and comfortable and relaxed. I always start at the head because I can imagine the feeling of relaxation flowing through me from the top to the bottom.

Here is another extract.

Bring your attention to your scalp, become aware of the top of your head. Feel a nice warm, relaxing sensation all over the top of your head. Now feel it slowly moving down your entire body, relaxing each part of you. Feel your forehead becoming smooth and softened. Let the relaxation spread more and more over the forehead. This pleasant feeling slowly flows all over your head, making you feel comfortable and relaxed. Now feel your eyelids, eyebrows and the muscles around your eyes: let them become heavy and sleepy and comfortable. Now become aware of all the many muscles in your face. Allow all these muscles to relax, so your face becomes expressionless and you look as if you're sound asleep. Even your lips part slightly and so does your tongue inside your mouth. Make sure your jaw is relaxed. If the jaw muscles are held tightly the tension radiates into the rest of our body, especially the head and scalp. Tension drains energy from us, and by simply giving our attention to each part of the body we can relax deeply. By being aware of the body, part by part and muscle by muscle, the entire body is completely freed of tension and stress. You feel loose, relaxed, soft and comfortable.

The exercise continues in this way, going through all the body so that you can release all the tension. At the end of the exercise you should feel warm and deeply relaxed, sinking into the chair or bed. In fact you feel so comfortable that it is very hard to do anything at all afterwards!

After deep relaxation you need to gradually rouse yourself with gentle movements and some stretching out. After 20 minutes' relaxation it will take another five to ten minutes to be fully alert again.

Relaxing the mind: visualisation

As an alternative to this sort of relaxation exercise, or in addition to it, you could try a visualisation exercise. The relaxation exercise should be done first, followed by the visualisation or some relaxing music. Visualisation is aimed at relaxing the mind and this is probably more important than relaxing the body. We have all had occasions when it has been impossible to sleep because of the thoughts going round in our heads. If you are able to calm the mind then this will enable you to sleep and it will also help you to free your mind from anxiety and to reduce the build-up of stress.

Ideally you should try to achieve both types of relaxation, and use them as and when they are needed. You will still need to take the deep breaths and quieten your breathing at the beginning, as in the previous exercise. Try to concentrate on the breathing and let thoughts drift in and out of your mind, but do not concentrate on any one thing for long. You could focus on something in the room if this makes it easier for you to concentrate and quieten your mind.

After your breathing is quieter imagine a place that you like to visit. It could be somewhere outside, like a garden or somewhere in the country, or it could be a room or an inside situation that makes you feel relaxed. Imagine the details, the colours or even the smells of this place. Alternatively, you could imagine yourself to be on a magic carpet that can fly you to wherever you want. You can then look down onto a beach or a lake or a village and imagine what you see below. If you find this hard to do you can buy recordings of the jungle or sea sounds to assist you until practice has improved your skills.

Here is an extract of a visualisation that I have used. I obtained this script when I was working at a community mental health trust running a relaxation course.

> You are lying on a beach in a safe, quiet cove. Settle into the soft, warm sand beneath you. It is warm and sunny, just the perfect temperature for you. You are feeling relaxed and calm as you look out at the calm blue sea. Just little ripples of waves coming in. Through the clear water you can see seaweed and pebbles and shells. Further out a boat is slowly moving along the line of the horizon and the sea is reflecting the clear blue sky with just the odd wispy cloud. You see a few birds flying overhead, and hear a few seagulls. You feel peaceful and relaxed, you are in the perfect place for you.

> Take a look around. What do you see? Perhaps you notice a cliff with a path running around the top. There may be people walking along this path enjoying the scenery, or other people on the beach quietly enjoying themselves too. As you look at the cliff face you may see birds nesting, flying to and from their nests. If you like, take time to explore rock pools full of sea life, filled with sea anemones, crabs and shrimps.

> Watch the gentle waves lapping over the soft, smooth sand. Can you smell the salty, refreshing air? The whole scene is peaceful. You are at peace, warm, comfortable and relaxed. You can stay on the beach and relax for a little while longer...

You can record this type of visualisation onto a tape or CD by using an extract from a book or devising your own scenario, or you can just imagine any place that is special for you. (You would obviously not use this scenario if water makes you anxious or you are worried about heights.) The idea is to look all around the scene and imagine the details. Focusing on this will help you to relax and will block out other thoughts and give you a chance to be peaceful and quiet.

Activity as relaxation

Another way of relaxing is to do an activity that you really enjoy. This will not achieve complete relaxation but it will help reduce symptoms of stress because it will take your mind off whatever is causing you stress. If the activity involves exercise this is even better as it will give you extra benefits. The next chapter explores the subject of work and leisure and the benefits they bring and also gives some ideas to help you achieve your goals.

A personal scenario

I first learnt meditation at a yoga class and this helped me to know how to relax. During each of my pregnancies I always had a period of deep relaxation in the middle of the day, just for 20 minutes. It really helped to recharge me. During my third pregnancy I learnt self-hypnosis, which is really just deep relaxation, and it certainly gave me a very easy pregnancy and birth. My third daughter was born in a few minutes. I had been so relaxed I had hardly noticed the contractions! I had a bath, went to bed and when I awoke at 5am rushed off to hospital and only just made it into the delivery room before she made her appearance!

I use relaxation if I need to recharge my energy, or if I am tense before an interview or a meeting. Once you have learnt relaxation it is always easier to notice when your muscles are tense and then you can relax them. You will learn to be aware of the postures of stress.

Key points

- Finding ways of dealing with stress can help you cope with rheumatoid arthritis.
- Learn to spot stress symptoms: physical, cognitive and behavioural.
- Relaxation techniques and yoga help to recharge energy and restore your health.
- Relaxing the mind is important too.

9

Work and Leisure

You never know what you can do until you try.

Employment is likely to be one of the most important issues for you, particularly if you are less than 65 years old. Work could be essential for financial reasons or because the job is important in its own right or both. Whatever the reason, it is often preferable to continue some form of work in order to have a purpose for getting up each day. Work always brings benefits whether it is for financial rewards, job satisfaction, social contact or all three. People often become depressed through the loss of the working role, and they often lose self-esteem and confidence in their abilities. The longer someone is out of work the harder it is to restart and this applies even more to people with rheumatoid arthritis.

The benefits of employment

A study by Reisine *et al*[1] in 1998 set out to test the hypothesis that 'employment confers a health benefit to women with rheumatoid arthritis'. Four hundred and sixteen women were followed up after being recruited seven years earlier from rheumatology clinics. Women who were employed had significantly better health outcomes as measured by disability, role function (carrying out everyday roles) and clinical status. The women who did the worst were those who had been employed previously but lost their employment during the study. The hypothesis was therefore correct and this study proves that employment confers health benefits.

Many young rheumatoid arthritis patients will be working when they are diagnosed, but according to research many will stop working very early in the disease process. This is in spite of the move to earlier medical treatment.

One study in Norfolk[2] set out to establish the rates of work disability in rheumatoid arthritis patients who were all employed at the onset of their disease. It was found that after two years nearly one third had stopped working. A study of 732 at St Albans[3] also found that 29% of patients stopped work because of the disease within five years of diagnosis. It is well recognised that work confers health benefits, yet many rheumatoid arthritis patients give up work early on after diagnosis. It is therefore important to know why people stop working, which people are most likely to stop and what can be done to prevent people becoming unemployed. I have looked at research to find out the answers to these questions.

Factors that help you stay in employment

The answers can be given in relation to personality and environmental reasons. They can also be given in relation to the type of work and the changes that had been made to the working pattern. Robinson and Walters[4] found out that workers who stayed employed usually had inside jobs that they enjoyed and were motivated to do. They had low absenteeism and they usually did not change occupations after the disease onset.

A study in the USA in 2001[5] found out that the significant factors for staying on at work were being younger, being self-employed, having a higher prestige occupation and having a higher educational level. The workers in this study also tended to work long hours and rarely missed work. These factors are all associated with the type of work and the characteristics of the workers, but some research has focused on the coping mechanisms that help workers to stay employed.

Research by Chorus *et al* in 2001[6] found out that adjusting job demands was the most relevant factor in reducing withdrawal from the workplace. The adjustments made included:

- limiting activities;
- pacing activities;
- being offered new training;
- encouraging workers to inform work colleagues of problems that they were having; and
- having an appropriate job.

These are all important ways of encouraging workers to remain in work. The following section outlines suggestions that may help you to stay employed.

How you can help yourself to stay in work

If you can be referred to an Occupational Therapist then he or she can be of assistance if you need an assessment of your general work pattern and work environment. You can then consider energy conservation, changing positions of work and joint protection in relation to your own situation. OTs may also provide working splints to protect your joints. These are useful for reducing pain by keeping the joint protected and stabilised during work.

The therapist may also ask you to consider changing the way that tasks are organised, or changing the work environment in some way. He or she could liaise with your employer if you wish or they may ask you to contact Access To Work (see below) to assist with the funding of alterations of the work environment. It is helpful to have the support of an OT if possible, but if not there may be someone in your company who can help you. You need to consider options for change in your work environment, and in the way that you carry out your work and the type of work that you do.

Access to Work

Access to Work is a scheme that was set up to enable people to stay in work. This scheme can be accessed at the Jobcentre Plus which is part of the newly named Department of Work and Pensions. It enables people to overcome various problems related to work. Examples of this are transport, equipment in the work environment and the facilities of the workplace, e.g. social areas or toilets. If, for instance, it is not possible for someone to drive to work or use public transport a taxi may be funded. Alternatively if a machine or a computer needs adapting then Access to Work could help with this. They may, for instance, fund a special chair or a different door entry system or an adapted telephone.

There will be an officer specialising in disability at Jobcentre Plus. These officers have training to assist people with disabilities to find a job and they can also liaise with Access to Work.

The Disability Discrimination Act

The Disability Discrimination Act should encourage employers in companies to make reasonable adjustments for employees with disabilities, such as adjusting hours, altering the job description slightly, making allowances for other staff to help out when there is a problem, etc. The Disability Discrimination Act states that people with disabilities should have as equal access to work as non-disabled workers. An employer must try to find an alternative job if the present situation cannot easily be adjusted to accommodate the worker.

Changing work

Sometimes, after discussion of the working day, it may seem more appropriate for you to change jobs and/or be retrained if this is possible. At the end of the day, health is the most important issue and serious consideration should be given to changing jobs if the present one is detrimental to your health and well-being. You may then need assistance with completing forms.

Completing medical forms

This can always be difficult for those of us who have disabilities or a chronic medical condition. Many people feel that if they mention the disability or illness they may not stand a chance of getting the job, and if they do not mention it then employers may try to find ways to dismiss them if they find out about it later. I have found that it is best not to mention it until the medical form has to be completed. At this point include the diagnosis on the form but add positive medical information with it on the form or in a covering letter. Obtain a good health reference from anywhere that you have worked recently, either in paid employment or voluntary work, and this will hopefully make up for the illness. Remember that it is possible to have good health when you have a chronic illness. Many people with rheumatoid arthritis do not tend to catch many colds or other infections to which other people are susceptible.

It is my feeling that the Disability Discrimination Act may be very positive in enabling people to stay on working for their present employers, but it may not be so helpful when new positions are required because employers could be afraid of the responsibility of employing someone who could turn out to be a liability. This is why you need the good health reference and you may also need further assistance to enable you to start a new job.

Starting work

If you receive a means-tested disability benefit (either incapacity benefit or income support for disability or the employment support allowance) then you will probably be referred to a disability specialist programme like 'Pathways to Work' or 'New Deal'. A personal adviser will help you draw up an action plan for your return to work. The adviser may refer you for a work preparation course if this is needed. In some areas there are also Condition Management courses delivered in partnership with the NHS to help people understand and manage their conditions in the work environment. There is also a WORKSTEP or Work Choice programme for those people who feel that they need a lot of support to return or start work. Access to Work can also be used for people starting a new job as well as for those wanting to stay in work.

If you are not claiming any benefits then you are not eligible for these schemes, but you may be able to use 'Next Step'. This nationwide organisation gives information and advice by telephone on jobs and careers. It also has a job website and information on writing CVs. Next Step can offer more in-depth interviews and support for people over 20 with fewer than five GCSEs at A–C grade and no level 2 NVQ qualifications.

Disability benefits

Working tax credit

If you are unable to find suitable full-time work and you have a disability, then you could be eligible for the working tax credit. This can top up your income if you have to worker shorter hours due to a disability. You will need to be working at least 16 hours a week and be receiving a disability benefit. You will also need to have received a work disability benefit like incapacity benefit or the employment support allowance within the last six months. Check the HM Revenue and Customs disability helpsheet or telephone for assistance.

The Jobcentre Plus may also be able to help you. This benefit depends on your financial situation. If you have a partner who is working, or if you receive an average or higher rate of pay, then you are unlikely to qualify. If you are single, or you and your partner receive low pay, then you may qualify, but all your income will be assessed.

Disability Living Allowance

Another benefit for people who are under 65 is the Disability Living Allowance (DLA). This benefit has two parts, a **care component** and a **mobility component**. There are three levels of care and two levels of mobility. Levels for the care component are decided according to the difficulties that you have with daily personal care tasks and meal preparation. The mobility component is based on the extent of walking disabilities, both inside the house and outside. DLA is only awarded to people under the age of 65 although the benefits will still be paid after you have reached 65 if you remain eligible for them after you are 65. People aged 65 and over may be able to claim Attendance Allowance. However, there is no mobility part included in this. Neither of these benefits is means tested. At the time of going to press all of the disability benefits are in the process of change. The government is proposing to replace DLA with a new benefit called the Personal Independence Payment. This will be a non-means tested, extra costs benefit which aims to help people with disabilities to live full and independent lives. The plan is to make this a more objective assessment and there will be a medical assessment for all claimants. It is not clear what exactly will happen but it is likely that some sort of points-based capability assessment will be used. The government plans to reassess all existing claimants between 2013 and 2016.

Incapacity Benefit and the Employment and Support Allowance

If your RA means you are unable to work and you are under 65 you may be entitled to the Employment and Support Allowance (ESA) This benefit is now replacing Incapacity Benefit (IB). ESA consists of two parts: contributory ESA that is paid on the basis of your NI contributions, and income-based ESA, means tested and effected by income and savings. The first 13 weeks of your application for ESA are paid at a basic assessment rate then after this, if you qualify, there are two different rates added onto this depending on your ability to work.

During the assessment period you will need to undergo a work capability assessment and this has three components. There is an initial test, the 'limited capability for work' test, that looks at your physical and mental health abilities. This test decides whether you are able to qualify for any ESA. If you are deemed capable for work you will not be able to receive ESA and you will be changed to job seeker allowance. If you are deemed to have 'limited capability' then you will need to undergo a second test, the 'limited capability for work-related activity' test. This decides whether you have a limited capability for work or not. This will also decide which of the rates of ESA you will receive. The final assessment is called the work-focused health-related assessment and this is carried out to find out what type of health-related support you need to help you move into work. The government has already started to move existing IB claimants onto ESA.

Pros and cons of benefits

The problem with benefits is that once you start them and stop working it is difficult to restart work, because the benefit system is so cumbersome and slow. If you take work and have to reduce hours or stop, it can take a very long time to sort the financial benefits out. The amount of benefit claimed (if it includes IB, DLA, Housing Benefit, Council Tax Benefit and Income Support) may be more than you can obtain by working. This is not ideal as it discourages people from trying. The government now recognises this difficulty and is trying to make changes. Anyone with a disability or long-term health condition may be able to receive a job grant and/or a weekly return to work credit when going back to work. The Job Grant is a tax-free lump sum if you have been claiming a work benefit for more than six months and are starting work of more than 16 hours per week. The return to work credit is a tax-free payment of £40 per week for people who have, or have had, a health condition or disability. It can be payable for up to 52 weeks but it depends on the amount of money you earn, the hours you work and the benefits you were previously claiming. Have a look at the government website for further information.

The ideal answer for many people with RA is to work part-time but the amount of available part time work is still limited so if it is just not possible to return to work then the only answer is to claim benefits and do voluntary (i.e. unpaid) work that is stimulating or useful and take up leisure pursuits instead.

There are websites on the internet for voluntary work and it is amazing how many options there are. However, funding transport can be a problem if there is no car available or you are not able to use public transport. You could also find out about voluntary work at the library or at your local volunteer centre.

A personal scenario

I have never claimed any IB because I prefer to work and luckily I have always been able to do so. I mentioned that at the time my rheumatoid arthritis began I was at teachers' training college. During the next three years I worked in a children's home and then went to college to take my 'A' levels. While I was at college I worked part time in various jobs.

During the next 12 years, whilst I was a full-time mother, I had four further flare-ups but I always intended to resume a career when the children were all at school. I never thought about giving up on work because of the arthritis.

Before my career break I had worked in many office jobs and also as a computer operator, as well as a housemother in the children's home. I had not been satisfied by these jobs and wanted to change my career pathway. In order to help with this I had studied 'A' levels and whilst I was at home with the children I studied for an Open University degree.

The actual diagnosis of the rheumatoid arthritis happened when I was studying for this degree (although by then I had had the rheumatoid arthritis for about ten years.) Luckily for me I attended Occupational Therapy at this time and decided that this was probably what I wanted to do for my future career. I set about achieving this by obtaining any job that would give me some experience in the right sort of setting. It turned out to be a job in an activity centre for adults with learning disabilities. I also visited my local OT departments and found out as much as I could about the work and the training. A vacancy for a therapy assistant was advertised in one of the departments that I had visited so I applied and was accepted. I really enjoyed this job so I decided to train full time.

All the time I worked as a therapy assistant I was careful never to take time off ill if I could possibly help it. I worked part time so this made it easier. I needed to show that I had a good health record because I was afraid that I would be turned down for future jobs or courses if it was known that I had rheumatoid arthritis. I was able to obtain good references concerning my health when I applied for university, and also when I eventually qualified and applied for jobs.

Occupational Therapy has been a good choice for me because it suits me better in every way than the previous jobs I have had. I have found the work satisfying (most of the time) and it also allows me to do a variety of different tasks. This is good for my joints. I drive to clients' houses to carry out the assessments. I work in the office doing a fair bit of telephone work and I also use a computer. After 20 years I now find myself needing to make another change in my life. The community visits have now become much more difficult for me and so I have trained as a life coach and I am presently working on developing this role. Life coaching and OT are similar in some respects as they both have a positive approach that enables people to improve their lives. I am hopeful that this will be very positive for me too.

Changing pastimes

In my leisure interests I have probably had to make even more changes. I have always loved music and used to play the piano. Early in my life I lost a lot of hand function and soon had to give up the keyboard. I then learnt the clarinet, but after 15 years I had to change again and now I sing. Hopefully my jaw will not seize up! I also used to enjoy wine-making for quite a number of years but now the demi-johns are too heavy and, because I used natural ingredients, this became too difficult because of all the chopping, lifting buckets, etc. Sewing and knitting puts too much strain on finger joints so they stopped many years ago. I also used to love sports and was good at athletics and racquet sports. I did keep up badminton until about seven years ago even though I was never amazingly good, because all the time that I played I had little or no wrist movement. I used to play by tactics and I could run quite fast, though I did not play competitively but only for fun. I have always swum regularly and although I am now not a fast, strong swimmer any more I do still enjoy gentle swimming as well as stretching out all my joints in the water.

Avoiding the downward spiral

It can be depressing to have to stop doing things that you enjoy and are good at but it is really no use continually getting upset about what you cannot achieve. It is necessary to find another way forward because basically you do not have any option. The alternative is to get more and more depressed and do nothing at all. It is then that you will enter the downward spiral (see Figure 17).

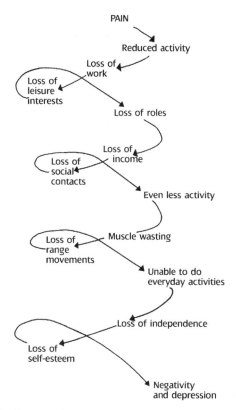

Fig. 17. The downward spiral.

People with rheumatoid arthritis can very easily enter this downward spiral. This is because the experience of pain and loss of function can quickly reduce the activities and roles that people usually undertake. Loss of roles and activities can then lead to muscle weakness, loss of movements at the joints, depressed mood, loss of self-esteem and self-confidence, fewer social contacts and reduced income if they lose their job. It is therefore essential that RA patients learn to adapt and find ways of achieving a fulfilling life and escaping the downward spiral.

Key points

- ▶ Carrying on working can have health benefits.
- ▶ You may need to assess your current work patterns and environment.
- ▶ Your health is the most important thing – changing your job or retraining might be necessary.
- ▶ Avoid the downward spiral by finding fulfilling ways of living.

10

Rheumatoid Arthritis and Relationships

Friendships multiply joys and divide griefs.

We have seen that rheumatoid arthritis is likely to bring change to your working life and to your leisure pursuits. There are also likely to be changes in your family life and in particular in the relationship with your partner. Having a long-term condition, particularly one that is so variable, is bound to make an impact on relationships. It is essential that everyone in the family, particularly your husband, wife or partner, is fully informed about the condition and the way it affects you, the person with rheumatoid arthritis.

If you attend any hospital appointments, or visit your GP, partners will be welcome, although if your partner works full time it may well be difficult for him or her to attend. Indeed, you may not want your partner to attend. You can, however, bring home information leaflets or books, and you can search the relevant internet sites and discuss the information later. Alternatively, you can leave information leaflets around for people to read. If family members understand more about the illness then they will have more empathy and begin to realise how you are feeling.

It is also very important that you talk about how the condition affects you because the books are general guides and not specific to you. We all have different problems. Some people have a lot of fatigue, others do not. Rheumatoid arthritis may affect the hands or it may be the feet or other joints that are most affected. Some people experience a lot of pain whilst others have more stiffness and restrictions in movements. The way that rheumatoid arthritis affects us is very different for each one of us and the way that we are feeling is different from one day to another. This is why communication is so essential.

Asking for help

Many people are reluctant to ask for help, yet at the same time they expect family members to know what help is required. This is a very difficult situation to be in. *No one will understand the way you feel if you don't tell them.*

I recently noticed a study on 'The negotiation of personal assistance by women with rheumatoid arthritis'.[1] This study highlights 'the complex nature of accepting assistance with activities of daily living' and it made me think about the impact rheumatoid arthritis can have on families and the way it has affected my own family.

Many partners do not know how to help you. They do not want to give too much help because many people with rheumatoid arthritis like to be as independent as possible. (It is much more positive to do the things that you want to by yourself and in your own time.) On the other hand, if they do not offer to help then it can look as if they are letting you struggle and are being uncaring. If they do help then they do not know whether to do the whole of a task or just a part of it. You must therefore talk about the help you need – *do not assume that someone can read your mind*. If you are given too much assistance you will become dependent but if you do everything yourself then you may end up feeling worn out and upset. Again it comes down to getting the balance right for you.

Of course, many partners and family members will work full time and if you do not work, or you work part time, you will not want to ask them to do too much. You may feel guilty or you may feel a failure. You could feel that you are being a burden if you are not managing all the tasks that you want to do. In the end it is still better to delegate if there is too much for you to cope with on a daily basis. You need to save energy and protect your joints. It is better for you to have a daily routine that you can manage without becoming worn out and stressed, than trying to do everything and ending up with a flare-up.

Generally people are happy to give a little help if you are patient and do not expect everything to be done instantly. One of the reasons that some people with rheumatoid arthritis sometimes do too much is because they want things done straightaway. It is difficult and frustrating to wait for something to be done and sometimes it also involves compromising on the way tasks are done. Still, even if the job is half done there is less left for you to do.

Making changes

Sometimes it can be a matter of changing household responsibilities. Choose the household jobs that you can manage most easily. For instance, you may be able to manage meals and light cleaning but not gardening and heavy cleaning. You may be able to do the shopping or manage the accounts and bills. Perhaps you can do ironing or washing up. Alternatively, perhaps you can go to work while your partner works part time. You need to negotiate to find out what will suit your relationship best and you need to do this by talking about it. Just because one partner becomes financially or physically dependent on the other one it should not mean that one or other person in the relationship is expected to do things they do not want to do. For instance, some people like their partners to help them with personal care but other people decide that doing personal care for a loved one changes the nature of their relationship so they decide to bring in a paid careworker or a friend instead. Both partners must be honest about what is happening in their own situation so that the best pattern can be established.

I keep emphasising the need to communicate, but remember this does not need to happen all the time. No one wants to keep on talking about rheumatoid arthritis on a daily basis – in fact it is negative to keep on focusing on it. Once you've discussed who is doing what, the whole subject can be forgotten about until there is a change. You can enjoy being together as a couple or family. Plan holidays and days out even if the rheumatoid arthritis is variable. *Do not let the rheumatoid arthritis stop you from having fun together.*

Rheumatoid arthritis and sex

Having rheumatoid arthritis may also affect your enjoyment and/or desire for sex. This can be caused by various reasons. It could be that you have a lot of pain and are worried that physical contact will increase your pain. Alternatively, it could be that your partner is afraid that he or she will hurt you unintentionally. Sometimes it may be that you just do not have the energy or inclination, especially if the only time you can get together is in the evening or at night time. Even if you have the desire, getting into positions that are likely to put pressure onto joints may be difficult for you. Moving quickly and spontaneously could also be a problem.

Another problem could be that you are worrying about the way that you look. Having painful, swollen joints or joint damage can make you feel unattractive. You may lose confidence and not be happy with your self-image even if your partner is not concerned at all about it. If you then avoid the closeness of a sexual relationship, or even avoid hugs and cuddles, it could feel like rejection to your partner. All of these difficulties can easily lead to both of you withdrawing from any physical relationship.

In order to prevent this happening it is likely that some changes will become necessary. It is important for both partners to explain their difficulties to each other. Try to make positive comments as well as pointing out difficulties. Tell your partner what is uncomfortable and painful as well as what is enjoyable. Talk about the way you feel, such as if you are afraid of pain or if you feel unattractive. Maybe you can make positive changes from this situation.

Having a bath or shower together can be relaxing and fun. Cuddling up together can also be enjoyable. You could try some massage together as this is very good for relaxing the muscles and reducing pain. Use this as an opportunity to try out new ideas. Some people with RA may experience some difficulties due to a dry vagina and if this is the case there are lubricating gels such as KY Jelly or Aquagel available from any chemist. ARC has produced a leaflet called *Sexuality and Arthritis*[2] and this may be useful for you.

It is probably a good idea sometimes to take anti-inflammatory medication or painkillers ahead so that you feel at your best when you need to be active. Obviously this removes the spontaneity for you, but it is nevertheless useful for making sex more enjoyable and your partner need not know ahead! Anyway, the rheumatoid arthritis varies for most people so it is always possible to 'make hay while the sun shines'. You are bound to have more energy some days than others, so make the best of it.

Taking exercise regularly will help to maintain your strength and range of movements. Exercise helps you to keep fit in all areas of your life including your sexual relationships. Incidentally, sex is good for helping us to exercise the heart and lungs and also for relaxing. It is very good for health and well-being and will certainly not be detrimental to your arthritis.

Rheumatoid arthritis tends to attack the smaller joints, and so the hips and back are less likely to be affected. This means that the joint pain and restrictions of movement that you experience will make less impact on sexual relationships. Yet having pain in your feet, hands, wrists and knees, the joints most often involved in rheumatoid arthritis, can still cause difficulties and this has been the case for me.

A personal scenario

My husband has had to put up with my rheumatoid arthritis for a very long time. The rheumatoid arthritis started when we had been married for just nine months. In fact he only knew me for 18 months without rheumatoid arthritis. Of course we did not know that it was rheumatoid arthritis then and so we hoped that the pain would go away and I would be back to normal. Even when I was diagnosed we tended to look on the bright side and just dealt with problems as they arose. I am a very independent person, and we are both problem-solvers and we try to work together to resolve difficulties. He is very supportive, but tends to let me bring up the difficulties, and ask for help when I need to and this is the way I prefer things to be. I think that I would feel guilty if I could not contribute to our household responsibilities and I do like to work to help with finances. So far we have worked things out and hopefully you will be able to as well.

I have had no wrist movement since my twenties and have not been able to support my weight easily except on my elbows. I have damaged finger joints and it is therefore difficult to use my hands. Sometimes my feet or knees are painful if pressure is put on them and occasionally my shoulders hurt. Luckily I have not often had fatigue and I am usually an energetic person and this certainly helps. I sometimes use Ibuprofen to take away swelling and stiffness. Changes have happened over a long period of time and this has made it is easier to adapt, but it has not all been plain sailing. I have often had times when I feel that I am not attractive and sometimes this still worries me. I try to do the best that I can to keep fit and healthy and to resolve difficulties as much as possible when they arise and this is the best that I can do. I am an eternal optimist and this is the way I survive!

Key points

- ▶ Living with rheumatoid arthritis can affect family life and relationships.
- ▶ Make sure people close to you have an understanding of your condition and needs.
- ▶ Find positive ways of dealing with sexual difficulties which rheumatoid arthritis may present.
- ▶ Ask for help when you need to.

11

Achieving a Positive Outlook

Most worries are future-based; they revolve around things that in most cases will never happen. (Wilson)[1]

I have written this book to encourage people with rheumatoid arthritis to begin to take more control of their life, by finding ways of solving their problems, learning about their condition and generally helping themselves to achieve a more positive outlook. In order to become more positive it is necessary to have some understanding of the psychological effects of chronic conditions. The psychological aspects are important because they can prevent us from accepting our situation, making changes and taking control of our lives. It is difficult for people to be positive when they are diagnosed with a chronic condition that has no cure. People are very different and deal with the diagnosis in a variety of ways but nevertheless some generalisations can still be made.

Dealing with the diagnosis

I started thinking about how I had felt all those years ago and then I began to realise that what I had experienced when I found out that I had rheumatoid arthritis were actually the stages of grief:

- shock and disbelief;
- 'Why me?';
- anger;
- depression;
- denial;
- seeking information;
- acceptance.

During my OT training we learnt about these stages of grief in connection with bereavement, but they also apply to other losses that we experience in our lives when we have a chronic, deteriorating condition. Having rheumatoid arthritis definitely feels like a loss because you feel that you will lose your future as an active, fit, healthy person. It is not what you had planned for your life. As well as the loss of health and energy, you begin to think of other losses. For instance, you may worry that if you cannot work you will lose money and all the things that it can buy, as well as losing your self-esteem and confidence. You may feel that rheumatoid arthritis will make you a less attractive person if you end up with deformities or swollen joints. You might also worry about losing friends if you do not feel well enough to go out and socialise. Going through the stages of grief is therefore a very normal thing to do, considering the uncertain future. We need to go through these stages to be able to move on and reach the last stage of acceptance. It is then possible to make changes and develop new skills and interests and generally get on with life.

How we deal with loss

Shock and disbelief

The first stage of grief is shock and disbelief and this will usually happen when you learn that you have rheumatoid arthritis. Alternatively it could be a relief if you were expecting something worse or had no diagnosis previously. Sometimes it is better to realise that there is a reason for the way that you feel. I felt upset in the first few weeks and months, and wanted to keep talking about it, which is the way I expressed my feelings. Some of you may act in a different way, by crying or by feeling that you do not really have rheumatoid arthritis and that it must all be a mistake.

Why me?

The next reaction is often 'Why me?' Why should I have to deal with this disabling condition? What have I done to deserve this? This is a very normal and understandable reaction and it is part of the second stage of grief. It is very reasonable to feel a certain amount of self-pity if you have a chronic condition with no cure, because you may feel that there are many things that you will now never be able to achieve in your life. It will also feel unfair to have to put up with pain – and very unfair to have the rheumatoid arthritis at all – and all this could make you feel angry.

Anger

There are many other reasons for feeling angry too. You may be angry because you cannot keep a job or obtain one. You may be angry and upset because you are not able to do all the things that you want to. Some people may feel annoyed that their partners or family are not helping them enough or that work colleagues do not understand. Anger is also part of the second stage of grief and resentment of others is also a part of this.

Depression

In some cases suppressed anger can lead to depression. Studies have found that the prevalence of clinical depression in patients with rheumatoid arthritis is higher than in that of the general population. Anyone with depression will be unable to motivate him or herself to get on with life or to make changes. It is therefore important to seek help early on if you find yourself becoming very negative about everything. Discussing problems and trying to find some solutions to at least some of them will help to prevent a deterioration of mental health.

Denial

Another common problem, which can reduce the effectiveness of treatment, is denial of reality or focusing only on obtaining a cure. Denial is a way of protecting yourself from unpleasant truths and future worries and it is also a part of the second stage of grief. It is true that too much information too soon can promote anxiety and fear, but denying to yourself that you have the condition can prevent you from getting on with life and making the necessary changes now. Although it is necessary to have some hope of improvement, awaiting a miracle cure or waiting for health professionals to produce a magical solution is counterproductive.

In any case there is no answer to the 'Why me?' question and there is at present no complete cure for rheumatoid arthritis. If you are a Buddhist or Hindu or anyone else who believes in karma, then you may feel that you deserve the situation that you find yourself in. Many of us, however, cannot answer the question in this way and therefore we need to try to come to terms with the situation as it is. There is no other answer. Rheumatoid arthritis cannot be attributed to diet or lifestyle or anything that you could have brought on yourself. It is important to remember that rheumatoid arthritis is not a life-threatening disease and symptoms can be improved. *A very good quality of life is still possible with a few adjustments.*

Seeking information
Trying to make sense of the situation and seeking information is the third stage of grief. In this stage you can do a lot to help yourself so that you can move on to the last stage of acceptance.

Acceptance
The stages of grief do not follow an exact pattern. Some stages overlap with others, sometimes we go back a stage or we do not necessarily experience all of them. Some people experience a stage of depression after the third stage because they cannot make sense of what is happening and or see any future at this time. Eventually most of us will move on to acceptance and begin a new future.

Becoming an expert patient
Discuss any problems that you have, whether they are connected to work, daily living tasks, social life, hobbies, family or sex life. Ask about medication or gain more information on the condition. Talk to a health professional, or a friend or family member. Look up information in books, on websites or in leaflets, or just keep asking questions. If you have problems at work, think about the changes you would like to make and discuss them with a manager or Access to Work consultant or both. Be proactive and do not give up. Having information will help you makes decisions and achieve goals.

The benefits of active coping

Seeking information is an active coping mechanism and many studies have shown that people who have active coping mechanisms feel less helpless, tend to exhibit fewer symptoms and generally have a greater sense of well-being. An investigation by Parker et al[2] in 1988 studied 84 patients with rheumatoid arthritis. The investigation looked at functional status, such as ability to manage activities, coping style, the activity of the disease and pain. Parker found that patients who coped by restructuring life goals had better functional status and psychological adjustment than patients who hoped for unrealistic solutions or engaged in blaming themselves for the illness. A study by Bendtsen and Hornquist[3] in Sweden examined clinical well-being and coping in 222 patients with rheumatoid arthritis. Those who had accepted the illness showed less guilt and tension and more endurance, and those who had decided on an active life showed a more positive belief in the future. This is important for good health and well-being.

Positive thinking

Another active coping mechanism is **cognitive restructuring**. This is the idea of changing your thinking patterns so that you interpret events and outcomes in a more positive way rather than tending to focus on the negative. If you are thinking negatively about a situation try to look at it in another way. Many situations and events can be viewed in a more positive light. You must see the half-filled glass as half full and not as half empty! Do not expect yourself to be one of the few rheumatoid arthritis sufferers who ends up in a wheelchair with many disabilities and totally dependent. This is called catastrophising. People who catastrophise believe in the worst possible outcome for their future and become negative in their thoughts. It is important that patients with rheumatoid arthritis do not catastrophise. A study by Keefe et al[4] showed that patients who catastrophised tended to have poorer outcomes in terms of pain, physical disability and depression.

Helpful support

A lot of studies have researched the importance of social support by close friends or family. Social support is about relationships with others and how these can improve your health and well-being. This type of support can be effective in helping to prevent depression. *It is not necessary to have a large number of friends, but it is necessary to have the type of support that you need.* If people are over-supportive they can take over all your roles and do everything for you and this is not helpful. It is actually detrimental because you are likely to become physically weaker as well as gradually losing your confidence and self-esteem. You will eventually stop being involved in your own life! The support that is beneficial is the type that can be called upon when it is needed. What you want will depend on your lifestyle and what you are able to manage.

Riemsma *et al*[5] in the Netherlands examined fatigue in people with rheumatoid arthritis in relation to the type of support that they received. They studied the levels of fatigue in relation to how people managed their support networks, the activity of their disease and demographic (population) variables. The result was that patients who took control of their support networks and could call on them when they were required had less fatigue whilst those with problematic support had more fatigue (problematic support is support that does not suit your needs). This shows that support is only helpful when it is doing just that, *helping you when it is needed.* This allows you to get on with your life in your own way. Social support must not take over your life and reduce you to total dependency.

What support do you need?

The support that is needed may take the form of practical assistance, or it may be listening to your frustrations and just being there for you, or it may be helping out with suggestions. Some people might prefer a therapist or counsellor when they feel the need to offload, rather than discussing issues with someone who is involved in the situation such as a friend or partner. It is really up to you to decide what suits you.

The support that you need will also depend on your physical abilities and the pain you experience.

Severity of disease is not necessarily the most significant factor affecting your physical ability or the pain that is experienced. Other psychological factors play an important part.

This has been shown to be the case in quite a few studies, including one by Hagglund *et al*[6] in 1989. Disease severity and coping strategies were examined to see if they predicted the degree of pain and physical impairments that would be experienced. The severity of disease demonstrated no significant relationship to the measures of outcome, i.e. pain and physical abilities. This shows that the way that you cope is just as important as the seriousness of the disease when it comes to predicting how much pain or loss of abilities will occur. *The best way to manage is to readjust life goals and your work and activities.* Always find a new way forward and look for the positive.

Being positive is beneficial for health

Being positive has been shown to be very beneficial for health. Martin Seligman[7] has studied optimism and pessimism extensively and he has observed that pessimists are more prone to depression and more likely to have poor health. Optimistic and pessimistic attitudes seem to be set early on in life and are the result of how we are made, how we are treated and what events happen early on in our life.

It is possible to try to become more optimistic by interpreting situations in a more positive way. Many events can be viewed in different ways. For instance, if you have failed an exam you can choose to believe that you failed because you were unlucky and all the wrong questions came up; alternatively, it could be because the paper was much harder than usual. It could also be because you did not do enough work or because you are not really clever enough to be doing this exam and there is no use trying again. These are all possible interpretations and some are more pessimistic than others. Optimists will move on and find a new way forward or a reason to be positive. They will try not to feel helpless or hopeless. The way to be an optimist is to make realistic goals that you can achieve, and to look at all the interpretations for a situation and use the positive ones.

Achat *et al*[8] studied optimism and depression as predictors of physical and mental health functioning. They found out that optimism is associated with higher levels of general health perceptions, vitality, mental health and lower levels of pain.

A personal scenario

Some people are happy to depend on others, but most people like to be as independent as possible. It is particularly difficult to request help when you are young. I can remember going to an Open University summer school when I was about 27. At this time I did not know that I had rheumatoid arthritis but I did know that it was very difficult for me to lift anything. All the tea and coffee was in huge containers and I used to try to find one that was nearly empty rather than ask for help. I also found that when I went shopping it was very difficult to ask for help because no one could really see that I had a disability – you cannot see weakness and pain. Later on, as my hands became more deformed, the opposite happened. People either tried to do too much or looked embarrassed or stared at my hands. I do not really have a problem with this now as I just ask for help if I need it and say 'no thanks, it's OK' if I don't need it.

Of course it is easy for me to be able to say this now because I have had the condition for over 30 years. It takes time to adjust to having rheumatoid arthritis or any debilitating, chronic condition. I have gone through many stages in my life. At first I ignored the intense pain and carried on regardless. Then my doctor gave me anti-inflammatory drugs but because he did not let me know that I had a chronic condition I continued to try to ignore it. Nearly ten years later I decided that I wanted answers and I asked for them. On receiving the diagnosis I continually needed to talk about it. I was quite angry at the way I was told. Everything seemed to be so very negative, such as things would get worse, I would lose the rest of my wrist movement, etc.

Over the next few months I searched for information, as much as I could cope with. I attended the OT department. I was given the time to ask questions about medication or talk about practical problems. I learnt exercises to maintain as much strength and range of movements as I could. I learnt about posture and joint protection and many other things that I have written about in this book. Mostly I became aware that it is possible to have a chronic disease but also be in good health.

Helping yourself

I have concluded my book with this section about psychology because I feel that it is definitely possible to have good health and well-being whilst having a chronic illness. In order to achieve the best outcome it is important to help yourself and take responsibility for your health. The medical profession can offer some assistance but there are many decisions for you to take. There are also many ways to help yourself.

First, you need to be informed about your condition.

You then need to keep yourself as physically fit as possible, so that your joints and muscles remain as strong as possible.

Thirdly, find work and leisure occupations that you enjoy and are able to manage.

Fourthly, look after your social contacts; friends and family are important.

Lastly, have fun and be optimistic.

The cards you have been given may not be the best, but there are worse hands and it's the way you play your hand that counts.

Key points

- ▷ Understanding the psychological effects of the condition will help you cope emotionally.
- ▷ You may go through a 'grief process', working towards acceptance.
- ▷ Become an expert patient – active coping mechanisms put you in control.
- ▷ Good health and a feeling of well-being are achievable.

Appendix
The Work of the
Occupational Therapist

Occupational Therapists, or OTs as they are known, work mainly in hospitals or Social Service departments or Community Health teams. They work with anyone who has a disability, whether this is a physical disability, a learning disability, a mental health problem or a combination of these. OTs use occupation to help their clients to restore or maintain their abilities or learn new ones. They enable their clients to carry out activities in self-care, work or leisure. Activity, both physical and mental, is essential for good health but to be of any value it must also be meaningful for the individual. Clients are therefore encouraged to contribute their own ideas for goals of therapy. The OT will then try to find ways for the client to achieve their goals (although these must be realistic) and in this way improve their physical and mental health. OTs will also help people to understand more about their medical condition as well as assisting clients to find solutions to everyday problems.

My initial contact with occupational therapy

I was referred to Occupational Therapy as soon as I was diagnosed, although by then I had already had the condition for nearly ten years. I did not know what OTs did but I did want to know as much as I could about the condition and so I thought it would be beneficial for me to attend.

During the initial period of Occupational Therapy I learnt exercises to maintain as much movement as possible in the joints of my fingers and wrists. I was shown special adaptive equipment and I learnt new ideas for working in the kitchen. This was useful to me as I enjoyed cooking and I had a family to cook for. I also learnt how to protect my joints to minimise further damage. In this way I was helping myself to maintain my hand function and strength as well as carrying on with an essential activity that I enjoyed. I also learnt about the disease and the medication available and I was given splints for my wrists. I found the sessions beneficial and I particularly enjoyed the chance to discuss any issues without being rushed out of the room.

A holistic therapy

OTs are trained in physical disability and in psychiatry. They also learn a lot of psychology in the three-year training course. This means that they are very good at assessing the whole of a situation. They will therefore look at medical, physical, emotional, social, intellectual, spiritual and environmental aspects. They will look at work, leisure and any issue that is important to a particular client. Financial aspects will also be included if these are relevant. OTs encourage clients to discuss any problems that they have in any area of their life. They will then try to find ways to overcome them. They will also assist people to reshape and reorganise their life if this is necessary. This encourages new potential. In this way something positive may come from a negative situation.

OTs as optimists

OTs are optimists and they build on the abilities of a client rather than dwelling on their disadvantages. After all, everyone has to deal with some restrictions in their life, whether it is their financial situation, their genetic make up or the hours they work. It would be rare if someone had a perfect life. It is better to concentrate on what you can do than spend hours getting annoyed and frustrated about things that you cannot change anyway.

We all live in a world where we expect quick fixes, but the patients whom OTs see usually have chronic conditions that do not get fixed. The only solution for any person with a chronic condition is to adapt to the situation and to maintain their health as far as possible. You can still have good health while you have a chronic illness, because good health is as much concerned with a sense of well-being as it is with the lack of disease. To achieve well-being you have to be able to have some control over your condition and your life. That is, you have to be able to cope. You will need meaningful roles and activities that you enjoy doing or get a sense of accomplishment from. If there is no meaning and nothing to enjoy then you will just give up and your condition will deteriorate further.

How OTs help people with rheumatoid arthritis

ARC produces a leaflet[1] about OT in which there is an outline of the ways in which OT can help people with arthritis. The examples given are as follows.

1 Giving practical advice to help overcome everyday problems.
2 Discussing your condition and how it affects you and what you can do to help yourself.
3 Making splints to rest or support painful or damaged joints.
4 Teaching you activities to help increase your strength or range of movements.
5 Teaching you techniques that will help you cope with pain.

This is a fairly good synopsis of the way that an Occupational Therapist works in Rheumatology, although as an OT I often feel that very few people understand that the main focus of the therapy is to enable clients to take control of their lives. This encompasses many things, like taking responsibility for the condition, making positive lifestyle changes, making informed choices about surgery or medication, choosing suitable work and activities, and enhancing general health by healthy eating and exercise. Ann Turner[2] in *Occupational Therapy and Physical Dysfunction*, says that the Occupational Therapist has a unique contribution to make in 'facilitating and promoting maximum function in daily living'. In other words OTs help people to be as active as possible in their daily living.

A–Z Guide to Well-being

Acceptance
This is about accepting your illness or disability but *not* about giving up. It is about accepting the position you find yourself in but moving forward.

Adapting your lifestyle
This is the key to achieving a good quality of life but also maintaining your health at an optimum level. It is about making changes so that you can still do many of the things that you want to. It is about finding new ways to achieve goals. It is about looking for alternatives that you can also enjoy.

Balance of activities
This is essential so that you do not put too much strain on any particular joint and so that you conserve energy for what is important to you.

Balance is also important when you have to trade off the benefits of medication against the side effects.

Choosing with care
Choosing correctly when you are buying new household equipment, tools or clothes is always essential. It can make the difference to being independent or dependent. It can also save the strain on your joints and prevent pain. Whether it's a new cooker, a new trowel or a new bed. *Try* before you *buy.*

Disability benefits

These can be important to allow you to be able to buy special equipment that you need, or care that you require, or it could be necessary to pay for an adapted car or a taxi fare. Having a disability always costs you extra money. Find out about benefits and enlist help to complete the forms at the Citizens' Advice Bureau.

Disability Discrimination Act

The final stages were completed in October 2004. As a person with a disability you are entitled to access employment, public services and entertainment facilities. Whatever disability anyone has they should be treated with the same respect as anyone else. Employers and people selling goods and services will need to make reasonable adjustments for you.

Employment

This is important whether you do paid work or volunteer. People gain self-respect and job satisfaction from working as well as gaining benefits of socialising. They feel more confident, and can maintain and update their skills. Work also gives us a sense of purpose and a feeling of being needed as well as giving a structure to the day.

Family and friends

Family and friends are essential. They need to allow you to be independent but should also be able to give support when it is needed. They can be there as listeners or they can give practical help – whatever is necessary for you.

Good posture

Being aware of your posture and maintaining good posture is essential because it will reduce the pain and the strain on your joints. Become aware of your own posture and enlist others to help you.

Heat

The application of heat to joints is also a wonderful way of soothing away pain. Buy a heat pack or have a warm bath or shower. There are also tubs of wax that you can use to improve the circulation of the hands, and thermal foot-spas too.

Hydrotherapy

This is a very beneficial activity that will ease any pain or discomfort in your joints and will help you retain a good range of movement of the joints. You may need a referral from a GP to attend or there may be centres that you can attend for a weekly session. Ask the GP or Physiotherapist. A jacuzzi works just as well.

Independence

This is about living your life and taking control of it. You do not have to be able to do everything for yourself to achieve independence. You can enlist some help as long as you make the decisions. Independence is very important for most people.

Joint protection

This is the way to maintain the joints as long as you can. There are three main concepts. These are avoidance of static positions, discouraging deformities and energy conservation techniques. Learn the basics and use them daily.

Keep moving

This is a very important tip because it will help you to reduce stiffness and pain and will help to maintain a good range of movements at the joints. It is important to use different joints by changing activities and positions.

Laughter

Try to find something to have a good laugh at everyday. It could be spontaneous laughter with friends or colleagues, a comedy programme, jokes in books or on the internet or an old comedy video. Remember laughter helps the feel-good endorphins to flow.

Medication

Good for controlling the disease, but always know what you are taking, and why, and find out as much as you can about it. Information is not always forthcoming and you need to know the pros and cons of any medication that you take. Medication should be reviewed and blood tests carried out regularly if needed. *Be aware.*

Nutritional intake

It is important to eat well so that bones and muscles stay strong and that your general health is good. Try not to become overweight because all your joints will have to work so much harder to cope, and so will your heart and lungs.

Occupational Therapy

A therapy aimed at helping you to maintain a good quality of life whatever your disabilities. Occupational Therapy emphasises the importance of keeping active with whatever is meaningful to you. This therapy helps you to problem-solve.

Optimism

Remember optimists stay much healthier and generally live longer than pessimists. People who catastrophise generally have worse outcomes for their health. Try to look on the bright side whenever possible.

Positive thinking

This refers to making changes in the way you think about things. If you tend to view situations and events negatively then you need to look at alternative ways of interpreting them. This is called cognitive therapy. There are courses and books that can help you. Changing your thinking pattern takes time and practice.

Questions

Always arm yourself with information from books, websites, health practitioners and anyone who can offer a useful tip. It is only possible to take responsibility for your health and make informed decisions if you have knowledge. Keep asking questions!

Relaxation and rest

These are both essential but are two different things.

Rest can be applied to any part of the body, or all of it, but the mind probably will not be included. It is certainly beneficial for the joints but the mind can still be working hard. Relaxation is about giving yourself a complete break from work or any ongoing problems and it certainly includes the mind. Relaxation is normally thought to include the relaxing of muscles, as in relaxation techniques, and the relaxing of the mind as in meditation or visualisation or guided fantasies. I would also include absorbing the mind in an activity you enjoy, even though the mind and body may still be active.

Specialised equipment
There are many gadgets available to enable you to carry on doing what you want to do. Alternatively, you may well come up with your own ideas. Remember, try them out first before buying.

Splints
Work splints or nocturnal resting splints can be provided by the Occupational Therapy department and will help to reduce your pain.

Taking responsibility
We have all become too dependent on expecting medical practitioners to give us a quick fix. We need to be involved in helping ourselves as much as possible with the support and guidance of the medical profession. Ideally, there should be a partnership, with both of us contributing in order to maintain good health. Consultants should be just that – someone to consult with – but the choices need to be made by the patient in conjunction with the practitioner.

Ulnar drift
This is the term for the way that the fingers drift when the wrist and finger joints are damaged. Practise the hand exercises and joint protection techniques to help you to control this and other deformities as much as you can.

Vegetarianism
Give this a try to see if the symptoms of rheumatoid arthritis subside. There is some evidence that it works for some people. However, we are all different and what works for one may not work for another.

Well-being

This is the term for the way that you feel about yourself and your health. It has nothing to do with the medical conditions you may have. It is the way you feel about your own life and health that counts.

Yoga

This is a very beneficial activity that will help you to keep the full range of movements in the joints, a supple body and strong muscles. It is also useful to relax the mind.

Zingiber Officinale

This is the Chinese name for ginger. It is thought to contain anti-inflammatory properties. It can be cooked and eaten in meals, drunk in herbal teas or taken as a supplement.

Tips and Ideas for Easier Living

In this new update I have decided to add in a new section. The idea arose because I realised that when I am in my own home or out in my own car I am almost totally independent. However, it is an entirely different matter when I am outside of my own home or office environment because then I can often feel disabled. It is the environment that makes me feel disabled and it's not nice.

There are many things that can be difficult for me. Here are some of my immediate thoughts.

- Hanging my coat on a hook and getting it off afterwards.
- Opening cupboards and being able to reach and take out items that I need.
- Opening and closing drawers.
- Turning taps on and off.
- Reaching plug sockets to switch on electrical equipment.
- Making meals or even drinks.
- Opening packets and cartons of all sorts.
- Lifting things.
- Reaching items on shelves and lifting them down.
- Going up or down some stairs and going up or down steep slopes and ramps.
- Getting off a low chair. I have to remember not to get on it in the first place!
- Having a shower or bath.
- Cutting up meat.
- Deciding whether to lock the toilet door. (I might not be able to get out again!)
- Undressing and dressing.
- Taking off a coat or jumper when I am too hot.
- Being able to drive a car that is not my own.

▓ Using some parking machines.

Most of these things are now not a problem in my own home as gradually over the years they have been solved one way or another.

In this section I have gathered together some tips and ideas that may be helpful for other people with RA. Some ideas I have used as a therapist, many I use myself and quite a few others have come from the members of NRAS. All these suggestions have been tested out either by myself or by other people with RA.

Personal care

▓ *Shampoo blocks/bars* are often easier to use than bottles of shampoo. These can be obtained from www.sosoapy.co.uk or www.lush.co.uk

▓ If you have difficulties when reaching *to wash under your arms*, use a long-handled washing up mop and place a flannel over it.

▓ Use a *sponge* to wash yourself rather than using a flannel because it's easier to squeeze out.

▓ Using a *bath lift, bath board or bath seat* can help you to use the bath if you are unable to get out.

▓ A *long-handled sponge or loofah* is useful for reaching all over your body.

▓ A *raised toilet seat* is useful for those days when it's really painful to get up and down from the toilet. It is removable.

▓ *Use bubble bath.* Then there's no need to clean the bath separately after use; just spray it.

▓ Buy *empty soap dispensers* and fill them with shampoo or conditioner if you have problems squeezing bottles.

▓ *Alternatively leave shower gel and shampoo bottles upside down* so that the liquid comes out more easily.

Drying yourself after a bath

▓ Try using a towelling tea towel, which is light, absorbent and will easily bend into creases and under arms.

▓ Use cotton buds to dry between the toes or use a hair dryer.

▓ Use a towelling dressing gown after a bath or shower to ensure you are dry.

▓ Get someone to stitch the two short sides of two bath towels together, leaving a hole for your head. This is useful when shoulders movement is limited.

Applying lotion

It can be very difficult to apply lotions to the body if you have damage to the hip joints or the wrists. Instead of buying a lotion applicator try a long-handled wooden spoon (smooth with no splintery bits) to do the job. Just squeeze the lotion onto the back of spoon and apply.

Brushing hair

If you have RA and you have restricted joint movement and poor grip it can be a painful experience to brush and comb out your own hair or your children's hair. **The Tangle Teezer** is very easy to grip and it glides through tangled hair effortlessly. It also gives you a relaxing head massage at the same time.

Cleaning teeth

- *Widening the toothbrush handle.* Put rubber bands round your toothbrush handle so it doesn't slip through your fingers if they feel stiff in the morning.
- An *electric toothbrush* is easier on the wrists and fingers and ensures teeth are cleaned properly.
- *Squeeze toothpaste out* by pressing down on the tube with your lower arm.

Miscellaneous

- Use light *plastic disposable razors* if shavers are too hard to lift and hold.
- Use a *make-up sponge* – it's easier on the skin too.

Dressing

- Wear *stretchy fabrics*, they are easier to take off.
- *Thermal fingerless gloves* are useful for inside and outside the house if it's difficult to wear gloves with fingers. It also helps to protect the finger joints from knocks,
- A piece of *ribbon or cord tied to a zip fastener* can make it easier to grip and to pull up and down.
- Use a *dressing stick* to lift clothing off the shoulders or to pull clothing up. It's also useful to reach things.
- Buy your clothes without *small fiddly buttons*
- *Replace awkward buttons with Velcro* (if you have to dress young children you may want to do this for some of their clothes as well).

■ *Leggings* are easier to put on than tights and are great with long skirts and boots.

■ *Wear a cape or a woollen wrap* instead of a coat. It is so much easier to take off and they are very much in fashion at the moment.

■ If you have trouble fastening bracelets and necklaces, try some with *magnet clasps.*

Lacing up shoes

■ You can buy *elastic laces* if it's difficult and fiddly to do up laces on your footwear. You can also buy *coiled shoelaces.*

Cooking and eating

■ *Battery-operated jar openers and can openers.* One Touch (the first widely available battery-operated tin opener) seems to be a favourite.

■ A *ringpull* is a useful gadget that lifts the rings upon cans and gets them open.

■ Try using *nut crackers* (the type with inside serrations) to unscrew small bottle tops.

■ *To open cream/yoghurt cartons* – cut down with a knife round the inside edge of the carton rather than attempt to peel back the lid.

■ *Cheese grater* To save the wrist strain that you get with vertical tower graters use a cheese grater that fits over a plastic bowl with a non-slip rubber ring underneath. The bowl also comes with a lid so you can store your grated cheese, carrots, etc.

■ *Wide-grip cutlery* is a must for weak fingers as there is much less pressure on the joints.

■ *Lifting dishes out of the oven* is easier and better for the wrist and finger joints if the dish is placed on a baking tray so that it can be lifted in and out with two hands.

■ *You can also remove heavy items from the oven* by placing a trolley beside the oven and lifting the dish with both hands onto the trolley. Then do a second lift onto the work surface (a metal trolley is preferable due to the risk of burning or marking a wooden trolley).

■ Use a *light tray* to carry cups and plates with both hands rather than struggling to lift them in your hands.

■ *Two-handled saucepans, frying pans and casseroles* make life easier and reduce damage and strain on the joints.

■ If china is too heavy, try lightweight *Melamine tableware.*

■ *Using a steamer* means that you don't need to lift pans of water and strain vegetables. If you don't have a steamer you could use a *cooking basket.*

- *Boil in the bag or microwavable rice* is much easier to prepare. No need to drain or ask anyone else to drain it.
- Buy an *electric mixer* for any baking/whisking.

Cutting and chopping

- *Right-angled knives* make chopping and slicing much easier.
- *Fiskars soft touch spring action scissors* are craft scissors with cushion grip handles for weak hands.
- When *cutting dried fruit*, e.g. apricots, use scissors, rather than a knife, to make the job much easier.
- Buy a *potato peeler with a wide-grip handle* or better still cook potatoes with the skins on.
- *Always keep your chopping knives sharp.* It is much easier to chop food and less pressure on the joints.
- Always have *scissors* handy. It saves a lot of frustration with packets.
- *Use a steak knife rather than an ordinary knife when cutting meat.*
- Take one with you when you go to a restaurant for a meal otherwise someone else may have to chop up your food!
- A *food processor* is a brilliant invention – it saves so much pain and strain.
- Use *garlic paste, garlic granules* or a bottle of concentrated garlic like very lazy garlic and very lazy ginger; so much easier than chopping.

Making drinks

Here are a few suggestions.

- A small *travel kettle* is great for making drinks for one or two people; alternatively use a kettle tipper.
- The *Breville Hot Cup* is useful for making drinks by pressing a button rather than lifting a heavy kettle. It can be refilled with a plastic jug.
- The *Dolce Gusto coffee machine* is also easy to use. Just drop in a sachet, place the cup under and press.
- Fill a kettle by using a *lightweight plastic jug* and only use a minimal amount of water.
- Always use a *mug with a wide handle* and not a cup.

Miscellaneous

- If you have a baby and use bottles, release the air by pressing the teat down. This makes the bottle easier to open.
- *Perching stools* are great for the kitchen when you need to keep getting up and down.

▨ The *freezer* is so handy to make up meals, then they are ready for difficult days.

Out and about

▨ If you wear *thin driving gloves*, contact with the steering wheel is improved so there is less need to grip so hard.

▨ Place a silk scarf or plastic bag on the driver or passenger seat of your car and you will *swivel with ease* when getting in or out of the car.

▨ *Insoles* can be useful for people with RA as they often walk on their heels and end up with pain at the back of the foot. The Busy Feet insoles are half insoles that cushion the heel really well and have a gentle arch support.

▨ An *umbrella can be used as a walking stick* on difficult days. Alternatively use a *ski pole*.

▨ Getting *petrol for the car* can be very difficult. Ask a local garage with more than one member of staff to serve you with fuel.

▨ *It's a good idea never to overload a bag.* Just keep to the minimum like a purse or wallet, keys, mobile and tissues.

▨ Buy a car with an *adjustable driving seat* so that your posture is better when driving.

▨ *Buying a new car* can be a real pain. Try the keys in the ignition, open the doors and the boot, try moving the seat forward and back and up and down, ensure you can use all the switches and levers and make sure you can manage the gears and handbrake.

▨ Buy an *automatic car*. It's definitely worth the extra money.

▨ A *shopping trolley* may be useful to save carrying, otherwise do your *shopping on the internet.*

▨ Use a *shopping bag with long handles* so that you can carry shopping over your shoulder or arm to save the finger joints.

Practical everyday ideas

Domestic activities

▨ *A wash-up sponge or washing-up brush* can be much easier to squeeze and wash up with rather than a cloth.

▨ *A dish washer* may be easier still; however, the warm water is therapeutic when you wash up yourself.

▨ When you are unable to reach and bend *an 'easy reacher'* is useful for help with dressing, reaching items in cupboards or on the floor and the hook at the end is useful to pull down blinds.

- When buying a *vacuum cleaner* buy a light model like a Bissell light vacuum cleaner or a lightweight Dyson.
- A *steam-ironing press* takes all the hard work out of ironing.
- *Dusting:* Use a *clean dish mop* as a duster for working in awkward corners and behind furniture. It saves moving heavy items.

Phones

- Have a *cordless phone with a speaker* so that you don't need to hold it.
- *Mobile phones:* A large touch-screen keyboard with a function called *Swype* means that you don't have to tap letters/words on screen, you simply swipe your finger across the keyboard and then the software (very accurately) predicts the word you're trying to enter.
- Use a *headset* with your mobile phone.

Electric plugs

- *Plug pulls* can be fitted to existing plugs so you can get them in and out of the sockets more easily.
- Some electrical goods suppliers will change the plugs on new items for *plugs with handles* free of charge.
- Change plugs on existing equipment that you use frequently to *'handiplugs'* plugs with the handle built in.

Wrist supports

- *Wrist support pads* can be comfortable and supportive when typing and relieve pressure on the wrist.
- To help reduce wrist ache, wear an *elasticised woollen sports wrist band* (sold in pairs).

For easing painful joints

- An *electric under-blanket* for your bed can be useful to soothe aching, stiff joints, particularly in the morning before you've got out of bed.
- You can buy *wheat bags that are microwaveable* to soothe joint pain, or you could make your own, by filling an old sock with wheat or rice and herbs and tying the end up.
- Use a *hot water bottle* on your joints in bed if they are cold or painful.
- *Therapeutic support gloves* help to reduce pain and swelling in the hands and make them feel more comfortable.

Miscellaneous

- *Folding trolleys or plastic boxes on wheels* can have many uses, such as carrying shopping from the car, or moving laundry in the house.

- Use *felt tips or thick, chunky pencils* for writing as there is less pressure on the finger and thumb joints.

- Use *wide-grip pens* or a *pen grip* around a thinner pen.

- Request *easy-open medication bottles* as the childproof ones are impossible to open.

- To *widen handles* use plastic tubing that will fit over the handle snuggly. If it is slightly loose apply some silicone adhesive (available from craft shops) and allow 24 hours to set.

- *For extra grip on rails in your bathroom,* cover rails with cycle tape, available in many colours from cycle shops like Halfords.

- *When you are unable to grip* ensure your hands are dry and also use a piece of kitchen towel to help.

- *Ensure washers are changed on taps* so they don't need to be turned off so hard.

- Change taps to *lever taps,* so easy to turn and available in all DIY shops.

- Change *door handles* from knobs to levers, they are much easier to open.

- *Key or knob turners* can be a good idea for Yale type locks.

- The *Magnetic Wand* picks up any screws, nails, drawing pins or metal bits that fall into corners where you can't easily reach.

- *Ensure drawers run in and out easily.*

- If bending down to pick up the mail is painful or difficult, fit a *letter box cage/catcher* to the inside of your door, under the letterbox.

- Use *chair or bed raisers* if you have to struggle to get up.

- When *buying a new chair* remember to measure the best height and seat depth for sitting comfortably.

Leisure

Gardening Tips

- When *planting seeds* you may find it useful to use salt/pepper pots to sprinkle out small seeds that are difficult to pick up.

- *Weeding:* You can reduce the number of weeds you have to deal with by covering the soil with a 5 cm (2-inch) layer of *shredded bark.* This excludes light from the soil and suppresses weed germination.

- *Pruning:* A *two-handed lopper* will give good leverage without much effort, protecting the finger joints from strain.

Three tips for digging

- A *border spade* is lighter and easier to handle than a digging spade.

▨ A *stainless steel blade* is better than a carbon steel blade as less soil clings to it making it easier to lift.

▨ *Spades with extra-long handles* reduce the need to bend.

Computer mice

▨ *Try out different types of mice* before choosing a suitable computer mouse. Some people find *a rollerball* is easier to use. *The Logitech Cordless Trackman* may be useful.

Books

▨ Use a *Gimble book holder* for hands-free reading or *lay the book on a table*.

▨ The *Kindle is an electronic reading device* and it eliminates page turning altogether. It also means that you do not need to hold the book.

Music

▨ Having a *pillow with an integral speaker* means you can listen to the radio at night without disturbing your partner.

Exercise

▨ The *Wii Fit and Wii Fit Plus and Wii Sports* are great fun for exercise in your home.

▨ Use a *dance exercise DVD* to allow you to exercise in the comfort of your own home at your own pace.

Dog walking

▨ Use a Crufts dog lead. It has a padded handle. Useful if walking the dog on a less good day.

Useful Resources

Books

N. Shone, *Coping Successfully with Pain* (1992) Sheldon Press.

E.C.J. Carr and E.M. Mann, *Pain: Creative Approaches to Effective Management* (1998) Institute of Health and Community Studies.

P. Wall, *Natural Pain Relief* (1997) Element.

M.C. Mason and Dr E. Smith, R.A. *Your Medication Explained* (2001) Sheldon Press.

C. Wetherby and L. Gordin, *The Arthritis Bible. A guide to treatments for arthritic diseases* (1999) Healing Arts Press Vermont.

H. Pain, L. McLellan and S. Gore, *Choosing Assistive Devices* (2001) Jessica Kingsley Publications.

P. Holford, *The Optimum Nutrition Bible* (1998) Piatkus.

M. Manning, *The Healing Journey* (2001) Piatkus.

P. Wilson, *The Little Book of Calm* (1996) Penguin Books.

Useful telephone numbers and websites

Adaptive equipment

Disabled Living Foundation. Advice and information about equipment for daily living. Tel: 0845 130 9177. www.dlf.org.uk

Organisations giving information on living with rheumatoid arthritis

Arthritis Research Campaign. Produces over 90 useful leaflets and carries out research. Extremely useful and informative website. Tel: 0300 790 0400. www.arthritisresearchuk.org

National Rheumatoid Arthritis Society. Promotes better services for people with RA. Volunteer telephone support network available for people with RA and also a helpline. Tel: 0845 458 3969 or helpline: 0800 298 7650. www.nras.org.uk

Arthritis and Musculo Skeletal Alliance. Campaigning to improve services for arthritis and raising awareness. Providing networking opportunities for groups to work together.
Tel: 020 7842 0910. www.arma.uk.net

NHS Expert Patient Programme. Self-help courses for people with long-term conditions. Tel: 0800 988 550. www.expertpatients.co.uk

Arthritis Care. Information, helpline and some local groups and self-help courses. Tel: 0808 800 4050. www.arthritiscare.org.uk

Help with pain management issues

Pain Concern. Information, helpline and self-help leaflets on a variety of topics. Tel: 0844 499 4676. www.painconcern.org.uk

Complementary therapies

Society of Teachers of the Alexander Technique. Find information on the Alexander Technique and a local teacher.
Tel: 0207 482 5135. www.stat.org.uk

British Homeopathic Association. Information on homeopathy and local practitioners, including NHS homeopathy.
Tel: 01582 408675. www.britishhomeopathic.org

British Medical Acupuncture Society. Practitioner listing for GPs and health professionals who practise acupuncture alongside their conventional treatments. Tel: 01606 786782 or 020 7713 9437. www.medical-acupuncture.co.uk

The Chartered Society of Physiotherapy
For information on physiotherapy and to find a qualified practitioner near your home. Tel: 020 7306 6666. www.csp.org.uk

Tai Chi Union for Great Britain, 5 Corunna Drive, Horsham, West Sussex RH13 5HG. Email: PeterBallam@aol.com

The British Wheel of Yoga. To find a yoga teacher in your area. Tel: 01529 306851. www.bwy.org.uk

The National Institute of Medical Herbalists. Information on Medical Herbalists. Tel: 01392 426022. www.nimh.org.uk

The Institute for Complementary and Natural Medicine. Information on complementary medicines, courses and practitioners. www.icnm.org.uk

Getting around

Public services and government website. Disability information on work, benefits, education, motoring and transport, health and support, housing and adaptations, leisure, travel and disability rights. www.direct.gov.uk

The Motability Scheme. This scheme enables people to use the higher mobility component of DLA to purchase their own car. This association also carries out driving assessments and provides information on adapting cars. Tel: 0845 456 4566. www.motability.co.uk

Disability information

DIAL UK. National organisation for a network of about 130 local information and advice centres giving information on all disability issues. www.dialuk.info

Disability benefits

The following telephone numbers and websites are useful for information:

Disability Benefits Enquiry Line. Tel: 0800 882200.
To make a claim for benefits. Tel: 0800 0556688.

www.jobcentreplus.gov.uk
www.dwp.gov.uk
www.direct.gov.uk
www.taxcredits.inlandrevenue.gov.uk

Employment

www.direct.gov.uk
    Help and advice for work and a job search facility
Remploy. Supports a return to work for people with long-term health conditions and disabilities. Recruitment service.
    Tel: 0845 6015878. www.remploy.co.uk

Access to Work. A scheme to help you and your employer find solutions to problems at work. You can be in work already or starting a new job. www.rnib.org.uk has good information on the 'Access to Work' scheme. Contact the Access to Work contact centre direct. Telephone numbers and information can also be found at www.direct.gov.uk

Nextstep. Gives advice and information on jobs and courses. There are local offices across the UK. Tel: 0800 100 900. www.direct.gov.uk

learndirect. Gives advice for getting a job and has a job search facility. Tel: 0800 101 901. www.learndirect-advice.co.uk

Education issues

SKILL. National bureaus for students with disabilities. Tel: 0800 328 5050. www.skill.org.uk

learndirect. Information on courses throughout the UK and on-line courses, as well as information on funding for courses. Tel: 0800 100 901.

Volunteer opportunities

Volunteering England. Find local centres for volunteer opportunities in your area. Tel: 020 7520 8900. www.volunteering.org.uk

Do-it. This website has details of volunteer opportunities in any area of the UK. www.do-it.org.uk

Leisure

AbilityNet. This organisation can advise people about adaptations for computers. Many factsheets available including *Rheumatoid arthritis and computing.* Tel: 01926 312847 or 0800 269545. www.abilitynet.co.uk

Carry on Gardening. The easier gardening website. Advice on layouts, tools and a question forum. Tel: 0118 9885688. www.carryongardening.org.uk

Tourism for All UK. Practical information on disability issues in relation to holidays. Tel: 0845 124 9971. www.tourismforall.org.uk

Miscellaneous

The Equality and Human Rights Commission. Information and advice on discrimination and other human rights issues. Helpline: 0845 6046610. www.equalityhumanrights.com

British Association of Occupational Therapists. Find an independent OT and check they are registered. Tel: 0800 389 4873. www.cot.co.uk and www.cotss-ip.org.uk

References

1 What is Rheumatoid Arthritis?

1 Mulherin, D (2004) www.rheumatoid.org.uk
2 Arthritis Research Campaign (2002) information leaflet *Rheumatoid Arthritis*
3 Baddley and Tennant (1999), in Bath, J *et al, Nursing Standard*, Oct 6–12; 14(3): 35–8
4 Arthritis Research Campaign information leaflet, as above
5 Hollander, J (2002) www.arc.org.uk
6 Marcenaro, M *et al* (1999) *Annals of the New York Academy of Sciences*, Jun 22; 876: 419–25
7 Haller *et al* (1997) *Clinical and Experimental Rheumatology*, Mar–Apr; 15(2): 175–7
8 Pollard, LC *et al* (2006) *Rheumatology*, July; 45(7): 885–9
9 Hampl, JS and Papa, DJ (2001) *Nutritional Reviews*, Aug; 59(8 Pt 1): 264–8

2 Pain and Discomfort: The Key Issues

1 Quotation from Autton, N (1986)
2 www.arc.org.uk (2004) publicity material
3 McQuay *et al* (1997) *British Medical Journal*, 314: 1531–5
4 Townsend, DJ *et al* (1999) *Rheumatology*, Sep; 38(9): 864–9
5 Berman, BM *et al* (2000) *Rheumatic Disease Clinics of America*, Feb; 26(1): 103–15
6 Campbell, D (1997) *The Mozart Effect*. Avon
7 Manning, M (2001) *The Healing Journey*. Piatkus
8 Affleck, J *et al* (1992) *Pain*, Nov; 51(2): 221–9

9 Pagnotta *et al* (1998) *Journal of Rheumatology*, May; 25(5): 879–85
10 Callinan, NJ and Mathiowetz, V (1996) *American Journal of Occupational Therapy*, May; 50(5): 347–53

3 Understanding Medication

1 Mason, MC and Smith, E (2001) *Your Medication Explained*. Sheldon Press
2 Arthritis Research Campaign (2002) leaflet *Pregnancy and Arthritis*
3 Ma, Margaret HA *et al* (2010) *Rheumatology*, 49(1): 91–8
4 NRAS Magazine (2010), New Year

4 Complementary Approaches

1 www.nras.org.uk information on diet
2 Volker, D *et al* (2000) *Rheumatology*, Oct; 27(10): 2343–6
3 Harwood and Caterson (2002) Cardiff University, www.arc.org.uk
4 www.arthritisresearchuk.org (2010) *Complementary Therapies*
5 Weatherby, C and Gordin, L (1999) *The Arthritis Bible*. Healing Arts Press
6 Siemandi, H *et al* (1997) in *The Arthritis Bible*. Healing Arts Press
7 Sands, L (1999) *Arthritis Beaten Today*. Vectropy Publishing
8 www.arthritisresearchuk.org on ginger
9 www.arthritisresearchuk.org on complementary therapies
10 McDougall, J *et al* (2002) *Journal of Alternative and Complementary Medicine*, Feb; 8(1): 71–5
11 Kjeldsen-Kragh, J *et al* (1994) *Clinical Rheumatology*, Sept; 13(3): 475–82
12 Palmblad, J *et al* (1991) *Rheumatic Disease Clinics of America*, May; 17(2): 351–62
13 Buchanan, H *et al* (1991) *British Journal of Rheumatology*, Apr; 30(2): 125–34
14 Arthritis Research Campaign (2002) leaflets *Diet and Arthritis* and *Rheumatoid Arthritis*
15 Mann, DL (2010) www.arthritistoday.org, on RA and food allergies
16 www.arthritisresearchuk.org (2010) on complementary therapies
17 www.arthritisresearchuk.org (2010) on complementary therapies

18 www.ehow.com (2010) Judge Abrams, *How to Find Research on Magnetic Therapy*

5 How to Protect Your Joints and Reduce Pain

1 Canadian Occupational Therapy Department (1991) The effects of an occupational therapy home service on patients with rheumatoid arthritis. *The Lancet*, June 15; 337(8755): 1453–6
2 Hammond, A and Freeman, K (2001) *Rheumatology* (Oxford), Sep; 40(9): 1044–51
3 Mcleod, L (2002) *Physio Footnotes*. painconcern.org.uk

6 Equipment and Adaptations

1 Nordenskiold, U (1994) *International Journal of Technology Assessment Health Care*, Spring; 10(2): 293–304

7 The Important of Exercise and Good Posture

1 Lee, MS *et al* (2007) *Rheumatology*, July; 46(11): 1648–51
2 Haslock, I (2000) *Journal of Rheumatology*
3 Hall, J and Skevington, SM (1996) *Arthritis Care Research*, June; 9(3): 206–15
4 Royal College of Physicians (1989) recommendations
5 Fentem, PH (1994) The benefits of exercise in health and disease. *British Medical Journal*, May
6 Turner, K (2002) *Star Treatment*, www.arc.org.uk

8 How to Relax and Manage Your Stress

1 Quotation from Wilson, P (1996) *The Little Book of Calm*. Penguin Books

9 Work and Leisure

1 Reisine, S *et al* (1998) *Journal of Rheumatology*, Oct; 25(10): 1908–16
2 Barrett, EM *et al* (2000) *Rheumatology* (Oxford), Dec; 39(12): 1403–9
3 Young, A *et al* (2002) *Annals of the Rheumatic Diseases*, Apr; 61(4): 335–40
4 Robinson, HS and Walters, K (1979) *International Rehabilitation Medicine*, 1(3): 121–5

5 Reisine, S *et al* (2001) *Journal of Rheumatology*, Nov; 28(11): 2400–8

6 Chorus, AM *et al* (2001) *Annals of the Rheumatic Diseases*, Nov; 60(11): 1025–32

10 Rheumatoid Arthritis and Relationships

1 Goodacre, L and Goodacre, J (2003) The negotiation of personal assistance by women with chronic arthritis. *British Journal of Occupational Therapy*, July; 66–7: 303–9

2 Arthritis Research Campaign (2003) *Sexuality and Arthritis*, information booklet

11 Achieving a Positive Outlook

1 Quotation from Wilson, P (1996) *The Little Book of Calm*. Penguin Books

2 Parker, J *et al* (1988) *Journal of Rheumatology*, Sept; 15(9): 1376–83

3 Bendtsen, P and Hornquist, JO (1994) *Scandinavian Journal of Social Medicine*, June; 22(2): 87–106

4 Keefe, F *et al* (1989) *Pain*, 37: 51–6

5 Riemsma, RP *et al* (1998) *British Journal of Rheumatology*, Oct; 37(10): 1042–6

6 Hagglund, KJ *et al* (1989) *Arthritis and Rheumatism*, Jul; 32(7): 851–8

7 Seligman, M (1998) Learned optimism, in Manning, M, *The Healing Journey*. Piatkus

8 Achat, H *et al* (2000) *Annals of Behavioural Medicine*, Spring; 22(2): 127–30

Appendix: The Work of the Occupational Therapist

1 Arthritis Research Campaign (2002) *Occupational Therapy and Arthritis* (leaflet)

2 Turner, A *et al* (1992) *Occupational Therapy and Physical Dysfunction*. Churchill Livingstone

Index

Made in the USA
Coppell, TX
22 February 2021